The Battersea Park Road to Enlighten
'A total delight. Isabel Losada navigates her way through the
eccentric highways and byways of the new age and human potential
movement with scepticism, humour and interrogative open-
mindedness. Candid, thought-provoking, sassy and very very funny.'
Mick Brown, *Daily Telegraph*

'Full of a crazy joy ... made me laugh out loud.'
Impact Cultural Magazine

'Humorous and refreshing.'
Canberra Times

For Tibet, With Love: A Beginner's Guide to Changing the World
'The world must be changed ... Isabel's story brings this truism
to life in a vivid, funny, heart-warming, delightful way. It is a great
read, a live teaching! I enjoyed it, laughed and learned a lot!'
Professor Robert Thurman, Tibetologist and Buddhist Scholar,
Columbia University, New York

'Isabel Losada is a 21st-century hero...someone who is changing
the world for the better and will make you want to, too.'
Harpers and Queen

'This remarkable tale of one woman's dedicated personal journey
captures the spirit of compassion in action.'
Lama Surya Das

'Fast, funny and inspiring too. Isabel Losada is a writer that
changes lives.'
Joanna Lumley

Sensation

Adventures in Sex, Love and Laughter

Isabel Losada

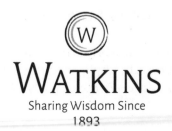

WATKINS

Sharing Wisdom Since
1893

This edition first published in the UK and USA 2017 by
Watkins, an imprint of Watkins Media Limited
19 Cecil Court, London WC2N 4EZ

enquiries@watkinspublishing.com

Design and typography copyright © Watkins Media Limited 2017

3 5 7 9 10 8 6 4 2

Designed and typeset by Clare Thorpe

Printed and bound in the United Kingdom

A CIP record for this book is available from the British Library

ISBN: 978-1-78678-093-5

www.watkinspublishing.com

Isabel Losada is the bestselling author of five previous books including *Battersea Park Road to Enlightenment*, which has sold over 100,000 copies in the UK. Isabel has worked as an actress, singer, dancer, researcher, TV producer, broadcaster, public speaker, comedian and author. She remains firmly committed to narrative non-fiction and swimming against the tide.

By the Same Author
The Battersea Park Road to Enlightenment
For Tibet, With Love
New Habits
Men!
The Battersea Park Road to Paradise

www.isabellosada.com

For P.C. without whom I would never have had the courage

for J.N. always

& for P.B. in appreciation

'An intellectual is a person who has found one thing more interesting than sex.'

Aldous Huxley

'Write what you are not willing to speak about.'

Natalie Goldberg

Sensation

Foreplay

My favourite joke:

'What's the difference between a golf ball and a clitoris?'

[Pause while the perplexed listener wonders how to answer.]

'A man's prepared to spend ten minutes looking for a golf ball.'

I entertain taxi drivers with this one and it always goes down well. Once the punchline was greeted with deadly silence and then the driver said, 'What's a clitoris?' He was winding me up. No, worse ... he wasn't. He really didn't know.

'You're having me on, aren't you?'

'No. Never heard that word.'

'Is English your mother tongue?'

'Yes.'

'Are you married?'

'Yes.'

'And you're how old?'

'53.'

'How is the sex with your wife?'

'We don't have any. It's terrible when we do. As you ask. Why am I telling you this? This is different from most of the conversations in the cab.'

'I'm going to give you a word.'

I wrote the word CLITORIS, like that, in block capitals on

a piece of paper.

'Here it is.'

I handed it to him with the payment as I got out of the taxi. 'Ask your wife if she knows this word. And if she doesn't please look it up and find out what it is. And what it does.'

This is all true. London. The 21st century.

• • •

Surprisingly Short Spring

Let's Talk about Sex

I am blessed with wanton curiosity. My favourite subject is happiness. I'm passionately inquisitive about it. I'm fascinated by what makes people enjoy their lives wholeheartedly – a job they love, service to a great cause, or even, yes, successful relationships. How many people do we know that have truly great relationships? Count the ones you know. You have to know them well to count them. I so hope you can use the fingers of two hands. Most people get stuck at two and a half. And why? Well, one of the reasons seems to be that at the centre of every relationship is a bedroom in which, often, hopes don't match libidos.

I've been writing about happiness for ten years and have never had the courage to write about sex. It's a bit of a glaring omission, don't you think? Many single people have a relationship with their own body that is based primarily on food and exercise. Many couples are completely sexually estranged. It's a tragedy of epic proportions when you consider the levels of pleasure that are potentially available and the levels of happiness, simple human kindness and connection possible. We are failing, sometimes, even to consider the delight of touch as an expression of affection. So, this year, I'm going to find out every single thing I can about sexuality and what makes it work and you can just sit back, read and hopefully pick up lots of glorious ideas. And before you decide I have the best job in all known universes … I'm not sure this will be easy. Not for me, anyway.

I was one of those single people who had forgotten that the body is designed for pleasure. I've been celibate for five years, apart from the occasional glorious stupidity. I had broken my heart over a man and I just couldn't find another one I wanted to get horizontal with. There is an expression, 'No one sleeps alone who goes to bed with a book.' And it's true. I travelled to strange worlds with Haruki Murakami, Kazuo Ishiguro and Italo Calvino. I laughed with Bryson, was educated by Oliver Sacks and fell in love with Rumi and Hafiz. I missed sex, but somehow these men were so enriching for my mind and my soul that I didn't care about neglecting my body. Contrary to popular beliefs I didn't become a wrinkled prune. I slept soundly and my days were full of other joys.

But then a new man came into my life, put the past in the past and brought even my sentences into the present. It's a shock. He is kind and patient, bides his time, makes me laugh and has a penis. Suddenly sex is back on the agenda. To have a man with a healthy sex drive in my bed again is challenging because, of course, like everyone I know, I'd like my sex life to be fabulous and I feel, frankly, that I have a lot to learn. I ask about the experiences of my friends and my readers, and I find that everyone seems to have a lot to learn. So, this is not a book about a relationship. This is a book, unashamedly and joyfully, about sex.

I'm not going to explore much of the alternative sex that

I know goes on out there in our cities. I have no interest in having sex with animals, plastic or groups of people. I have no interest in being tied up for hours by a complicated series of Japanese knots, being suspended upside-down, or whipping men who are crying out, 'Please punish me!' I know that women, somewhere not far from us, are being turned on by attaching cords to piercings in impressive places. I wish all consenting adults joy, but I won't be doing any of that. Call me old-fashioned.

I'm delighted by the idea of finding lots of ways to make sex wonderful. I hope that most of what I learn will also be useful to you whatever your situation. I'm writing about sex between one man and one woman because that's where I'm at myself. This kind of sex is what is known in the sexuality world as 'vanilla'. I assume it's called that coz it's uncomplicated and – as with ice cream – the best.

After all the 'spiritual work' I've done (see previous books for more information than is necessary for anyone) there is no way that I can settle for a bad sex life. The new man is offering me the possibility of a good sex life but I find that five years of celibacy and lots of bad sex in previous years has left me as lost and confused as most women I talk to.

In my spiritual life and in relation to others I know how to be – kindness and compassion as a philosophy serve me well. Now the spiritual has to join the sexual in a whole new way. They are not to be housed in different parts of my body and soul. Everyone that has a sex life wants a good sex life so ... I'm going to make pleasure a priority and I'll be encouraging you to do the same. There will be ideas in these pages that you can contemplate, consider and create – joyfully I hope – in your own bedroom.

And we'll have fun. Sex isn't a subject to be taken too seriously. We have a huge capacity for pleasure, as well as for love and the ability to make babies. So, please read with a pencil. Underline things, cross things out and find me on Facebook. Write to me, as I'm sure that I'll be learning about all this for the rest of my life.

We are calling my boyfriend 'T'. Not because he wouldn't have been perfectly happy for me to use his name but because we don't want to be the cause of anyone getting their knickers in a twist.

There is nothing so shocking, it seems, as having sex with a consenting adult with whom you are in a relationship. If we just open the bedroom door and look inside.

The State We're In

In *The Art of Sexual Ecstasy*, which Margo Anand published in 1989, she writes that a survey taken at that time questioned 90,000 women about their sex lives and asked whether they would rather be 'cuddled and held tenderly' or have sexual intercourse. Sixty-four thousand said they would rather be held tenderly and not have intercourse at all. Do you think the figure would be higher now or lower?

Somehow the subject of pleasure for women still isn't discussed. The clitoris for example ... If you take even a quick look at Wikipedia you'll be told that the clitoris is 'the primary anatomical source of human female sexual pleasure' (we'll be exploring that one later) and offered several scholarly articles to back up this statement. Press the link to the most recent of the articles and you'll be told 'the clitoral glans is very hard to find'. The article also informs us that 'more education about the clitoris' is widely necessary and would alleviate the 'social stigma' that still surrounds the subject of women's pleasure. There is a stigma, still, around the subject of pleasure for women? OK, so let's focus on that then.

The information revolution has made many matters worse rather than better as misinformation spreads fast, especially when someone has a product to sell. Men are now being convinced by online nonsense that their penis can never be long enough, wide enough or hard enough. And from the letters that I receive it seems to me that women are STILL worried that if they are not having multiple orgasms and screaming with pleasure then they are somehow failing. Heaven help young girls in their teens and 20s when their new boyfriends have watched Internet porn and expect women to respond the way the porn models do. And we have to feel very sorry for the boys who feel that they have to produce a performance – without ever knowing that what they are watching online is absurdly unrealistic. Apparently, in the US only 13 states require that sex education is medically accurate. (What on earth are they teaching if it's not medically accurate?) According to Peggy Orenstein's book *Girls and Sex* (2016), a recent US study found that after a 'hook-up' (which is defined as a one-night stand which can involve intercourse, oral or anal sex, but is usually only the woman going down on the man and not the other way around) 82% of men are glad they hooked up whereas only 57% of women are similarly happy. It seems that when mothers talk to their children about sex they concentrate on the risks and the dangers, while many fathers just joke and avoid the subject completely. Girls and young women lack even simple assertiveness skills in the area of sex.

Even older women still feel inadequate unless they are orgasmic during penetration and so lots of girls and women are still pretending. Somehow news that only a small minority of women are able to achieve orgasm easily through penetration alone seems to have been hidden in the small print. So the cry 'something is wrong with me' still echoes off the agony columns, one of the only places women go for sexual advice despite the fact that the columnist may have less than 400 words to answer. I've written a sex advice column myself and I can tell you that there is not much room for subtlety. The success of *Fifty Shades of Grey* illustrates how huge the need and the interest in sexuality is, while that series of books made the situation worse rather than better. It's all up to the man is it? The woman's pleasure? I don't think so.

For men, the result of the absurd performance pressure brought about by the porn industry is more impotence. Penises are staying down as divorce graphs are still going up. A Viagra pill doesn't make it all better. And while men are prescribed Viagra – often a woman's lack of interest in sex is considered normal. For some couples the bedroom may be the happiest place in their lives but I think it's fair to guess that they probably don't make up the majority of the population.

You'd think we just need more hippies, but in alternative cultures the situation in bedrooms isn't much better. The famous separation of spirituality and sexuality permeates every aspect of our society, and sexuality is often seen as either an obsession or feared and perceived as an enemy.

Historically, some would argue that there was no division in Christianity until St Augustine came along and ruined it all. The monotheistic God of the Judaeo-Christian tradition had created sex after all and, like everything in His/Her creation, had presumably created pleasure for the sake of – well – pleasure. Just as we can enjoy food and drink, we can enjoy sex. But the two fell out suggesting that if you wanted to explore the spiritual you needed to leave the sexual alone or keep it for the creation of babies. The position of sexuality in the Islamic world is also ... well, how would we put this? Often not a happy one?

In India, the situation is slightly better. Not a lot. There are three major traditions. The first is Vedanta, which teaches us that the external universe is unreal and the only reality is the absolute uncaused Cause/Consciousness/Source (pick your own noun, but use 'God' with care). The mind is the creator of reality and the body is part of the great illusion. For this reason, many of the great masters of this tradition, like Ramakrishna and Ramana Maharshi, show such a total disregard for looking after their bodies that they end up being carried off by cancer at an unnecessarily young age. This tradition is alive and well today in the form of Advaita, one of the branches of Vedanta, and experienced through teachers including Mooji and Eckhart Tolle. Tolle's books, which are basically a clear teaching of ancient Vedanta beliefs, were so phenomenally successful in America that Tolle was given his own TV channel – which I heard was a gift from Oprah Winfrey. But Advaita does not have, at the core of the teachings, any celebration of sexuality. The body is, at worst, linked to pain and, at best, considered irrelevant since it will age and then we will be parted from the temporary meat package that we walk around in.

Then there is Buddhism. In the way most Buddhist traditions are understood and taught today, sexuality is most often linked with craving which is one of the hindrances to enlightenment. Anyone mindful should at least avoid any form of sexual misconduct and the desire for sex. Full-time disciples of Buddha were required to be strictly celibate and our two best-known Buddhist teachers, His Holiness the Dalai Lama and Thích Nhat Hanh, are both celibate. Any serious student of Buddhism should neither desire nor be attached to sexual pleasure. His Holiness the Dalai Lama has said that the highly mystical practices of sexual yoga in the Gelug School of Tibetan Buddhism should be practised purely as visualizations. Thích Nhat Hanh has made famous the teaching that when we are drinking tea we must be aware that we are drinking tea. But, although I know he would say that the same principles apply whatever you are doing – as a celibate, understandably, he never taught about sex. All those profoundly spiritual nuns, monks and spiritual teachers from many traditions that I have met – are celibate. Some whom I've not met – other well-known spiritual teachers who are not celibate – rarely, if ever, speak about sexuality. They are very quiet on the subject. In short, there is not a lot of naked dancing, ululating and making love under the moon going on in most current spiritual practice.

And you can see why. Do I really want to write about this, you may ask? I mean, isn't it, like – private? The simple answers are – 'I don't know' and 'yes'. It would be so much easier to learn all this in private and write a book on lionfish. But this subject is long overdue. In the past I have not had a partner with T's courage. An honest man who is prepared to admit that he, like me, doesn't know it all. He and I have both been married; we've both had children. We have both had some sexual relationships that have been good and some bad. We both know very little.

'Hold on a minute ...' T interjects when I read this back to him. 'Who says I know very little?'

'Well, relatively, surely you must acknowledge that you know very little?'

'Compared to what?'

'Compared to all that there is to know.'

'I suppose. Relative to the sum total of the knowledge about human sexuality, then, yes, I know very little.'

'OK then.'

I proceed ...

• • •

The larger part of me would love to keep what I learn in the beautiful privacy of my velvet relationship, shielded behind curtains and protected by locked doors; or write dry factual information while keeping myself hidden. But this is not what I do as those of you that have read my previous books know. So, if I get accused of, well – heaven knows what I'll be accused of in broaching this subject material – I'll just do my best to dodge any of the sundry opinions that may come my way. If, as the spiritual teachers proclaim, the identity itself is illusory, then I don't have to worry about either praise or attack do I? I'll become a duck, attempt to appear serene on the surface, let much slide off my back like water and paddle like crazy under the surface.

I have so much I need and want to learn myself and I know, from letters that I receive, that there is much unhappiness and lack of connection out there in bedrooms. As I'm in the fortunate and privileged position of being able to learn, which is more selfish – to learn and lock my own bedroom door or to learn and share what I learn with you? So, I'm taking this on as my job for a while.

'But what about T?' I hear you asking me. 'How does he feel about this?' Well, this was his suggestion. Honestly. I was amazed. He said that, as this was an area we were exploring, why not write about what I learn? So I not only have his consent, I have his interest and his active enthusiasm. Good for him. I don't know many men that would have this courage. But I'm going to keep him out of this as much as possible just the same.

• • •

I've been asking questions on social media and inviting private responses from readers and friends.

This morning I read:

'I'm sure there is something wrong with me. Maybe I need to see a therapist.'

'Sex is fine for me with no orgasm ... I suppose.'

'I have great sex with my lover – just lousy sex with my wife.'

'The sex is much better with my lover than with my husband.'

So, just one day after committing to this project I've seriously decided I don't want to write this. How about a tome on the international economic situation? A series of mystical cards on the Tarot (channelled, preferably, by some higher being so I'm not responsible for bad grammar). A series of hand-stitched cloth artworks on the joys of flowers found in the works of Proust? How about a book on any sodding subject apart from this one? The answers to simple questions like 'How is your sex life?' keep arriving:

'The quality of my sex life has gone down with my husband since we got married.'

And more messages,

'My husband left me because he said he could give his girlfriend more pleasure.'

'Orgasm is all in the mind, isn't it?'

'I think there is something physically wrong with me.'

'I have to admit that since my son was born four years ago, I've had sex with my husband twice.'

'I'm fed up with all his pushing and shoving. I just fake

it so he feels that he can finish.'

Alternatively, there is a kind of smugness as if the ability to have good sex is some kind of personal success.

'I've been having G-spot vaginal orgasms all my life.'

'A man's only got to play with my breasts and I can come.'

'I met a man in a tantra workshop and I came just looking at him. We were both fully clothed.'

'I can orgasm just by having the man pull my ear and kiss my neck.'

'No woman has ever faked anything with me.'

Strangely I've never heard, 'Lots of the women I have sex with exaggerate their pleasure and fake their orgasm.'

The difference between the two lists and the amount of pain versus the amount of pleasure fills me with a kind of apoplectic rage. How is it that when there is so much information many people know so little and suffer so much? How is it that so many men, who want nothing more than to please the women that they love, don't know how to? How is it that so many women seem to suffer but feel helpless to do anything about it? Why doesn't everyone wise up a bit? Why are so many people watching cat videos and then having bad sex?

As you can see – I get a little passionate about this.

I ask on my Facebook page: 'What books about sex have both men and women read?' One man writes – 'I read a book called *Sex and Boys* when I was a teenager.' But, of course, he hasn't read anything since. The myth persists – we are all supposed to be perfect lovers 'instinctually'. Sheesh. This myth has got to go. A human body, or at least a woman's arousal and orgasm, is complicated and the factors that go to create these stigmatized pleasures are, I radically suggest, worth a little study. And learning how to really please your partner and please yourself too is great research.

Hey – the subject we're exploring here is PLEASURE!

• • •

Maybe one reason that more people don't learn about this area is that there are so many industries based on befuddling us. I just typed 'sex advice' into Google and have been offered 317,000,000 suggestions. Nothing even vaguely useful like suggesting people ask themselves, 'What sensation am I feeling?' The top one is, '10 Sex Tips Inspired by *Game of Thrones*.' Then I began to rend my clothes and dance naked in my garden. No, not really. But I felt like it.

OK, I want to avoid the ridiculous. I really want to learn about sexuality in a serious and dedicated way. I know that there is a source of traditional knowledge. There is an area that stands outside the sex industry, outside porn, outside most of what we know about when we think about sex, and outside the religious traditions that divide the soul, the body and my local archery class. It is a spiritual tradition, not widely understood but which is woven through much Tibetan Buddhism and Hindu thought.

Yes, you know, don't you? It's the tantric tradition; the one and only tradition in which sexuality and spirituality are one. So I'm going to start this journey with learning a little bit about what is now promoted as 'tantric sexuality'.

Tantric Sex Workshops for Women Only?

I thought I'd start with an all-women's tantric sex workshop even though any kind of women's work scares me. I have these terrible images of us being carried off to the woods by large groups of very well-endowed women with gold teeth and lots of nose rings and informed that I have to masturbate in front of them all or the development of my sexuality will be eternally doomed. I have never heard of a workshop where this happens but it would be just my luck to end up in one.

Even the thought of the conversations we may be having is slightly terrifying. What will we be talking about? Maybe there will be a competition? 'Sexual failures I've had. Major disasters with lovers. Memories I'd rather not have.' I have a few of those. I may as well confess now – it's easier to talk to you. After all, you are just my reader. You're not actually a living person, sitting in front of me with empathetic eyes and weeping silently. I don't mind talking to you. OK – so a few of my worst sexual misadventures.

Some of the worst sex I'd ever had was with one of the best-looking men I've ever slept with. A sportsman, an Adonis, he was so good-looking and so perfect that when he took his clothes off I felt as if I'd won him in a raffle. But as soon as he got horizontal it was as if he just wanted to get everything over as soon as possible. I'm not averse to a quickie sometimes but this was almost rudimentary. Zero 'foreplay' (terrible word that suggests it's just a preamble to intercourse – whereas with a good lover everything is part of making love) then past the finish line before I was even in the running. Maybe it was my fault and he was put off by the fact I don't have the body of a model. But he must have noticed that while I still had my clothes on. I wasn't upset; I was stunned. So much so that I didn't even raise an objection. I simply didn't know what to say. I don't know what deeply sensual experience my absurdly optimistic sub-conscious mind had anticipated but whatever it was, it was purely fictional. It's an old mistake to assume that a great body will mean a great lover. But it's not true, of course. Despite what the entire advertising industry tells us every day.

There was a man I slept with only once. He'd been a friend for some time and shortly after my marriage broke up I went to him one night for a little love and comfort. Instead we ended up having sex and he made animal noises – no, I don't mean he made sounds that were loud and wild and free, he deliberately, consciously, when he was having intercourse, made noises like a dog, then a pig, then a donkey, a horse or whatever. I'm happy to say I've forgotten the order and the details so I can spare you this information. I remember I wanted to stop and say 'What ARE you doing? Are you SERIOUS?' But he evidently was and became very carried away in his verbal expression of excitement – or something. Perhaps if we'd been in hay I could've got a little more into it. Somehow my inner dromedary remains suppressed.

And I had a Chinese boyfriend. Not Westernized at all. As you may know, there is an ancient belief in Asia, still observed by some Chinese men, that it is bad for a man to orgasm more than once a week. This would have been fine had we not been young and in love and having sex all the time. I remember distinctly him lying on top of me, with no penetration, sort of having sex with the air instead of my body, in some attempt to both be aroused and not aroused all at the same time. It was intimate but, you'll not be surprised to hear, predictably unsatisfying for us both. I now know that we had seriously misunderstood the ancient teachings. Whatever we were doing was certainly not what the sexually enlightened ancients had intended. Couples are probably making similar absurd errors of interpretation all across China still. In Tibet, meanwhile there are still women with more than one husband. And women there, who work in the fields and dig roads, sing while they work. But I digress.

I've never been a woman who picks up men in bars and takes them home for 'no strings attached' sex. I've always regarded women who can do this with a mixture of fascination, bewilderment and admiration. If an unknown man said to me, 'Get your coat you've pulled,' I'd just laugh and run the other way. To have sex with strangers you must have to be so totally uninhibited and have a kind of sexual confidence that is totally unknown to me. It's scary enough sleeping with people you know well. I've always wanted to know someone and even – er – to love them, before getting naked with them. I'd have a trouble even showering with a stranger, so how does anyone get naked and under the sheets? Did I miss something really obvious? Now I'm writing this I'm questioning everything about my sex life. I want to feel, at least, HUGE affection for someone before being so supremely intimate or sharing my morning coffee with them.

I began my sex life living with a man for two years, before we made a predictable mistake and got married. It was a marriage that, although happy in some ways, was a traditional disaster sexually, which was not my young husband's fault any more than it was my own. We had lots of sex, which was great for him, and I formed habits of not caring about my own pleasure. This experience between heterosexual couples, where women's pleasure is viewed almost as an optional extra, is encouraged by many cultures. In the church and in many religious contexts the subject isn't discussed at all and it's certainly not on the curriculum in our schooling system. (Or, at least, I've never heard sermons or school lessons in praise of sexual pleasure.) In terms of sex for procreation we were OK and I'm eternally grateful to my ex for giving me our beautiful daughter, but in most other ways we were so incompatible we couldn't have agreed on how to make a pizza. But we stayed together for seven years. As you do.

By the time we split up we both thought I was broken or defective. Divorce is such a wonderful and liberating institution. Really, people should have divorce parties. We celebrate the end of a life with thanksgiving parties, why do we not celebrate the end of a relationship? Partners could give speeches and say, 'I'd particularly like to thank you for the sex we had under that tree once on holiday in Greece.' And everyone could stand around, drink champagne, applaud and then tie cans on the back of cars before the couple drive off joyfully in opposite directions. All you would need to achieve this would be for both partners to tell the truth, 'Darling this has been great but I can't do this any more. Please release me. Let me go.' Burst into song if necessary.

As Paul Simon says, 'There must be 50 ways to leave your lover.' But I digress again. I was talking about my inability to master one-night stands. I'm not knocking this experience if that's really what both partners want. But I can count mine on one hand. I have always had this desire to associate love with sex and, in a rather predictable way, to want something more: emotional connection, intellectual connection, spiritual connection – all that stuff. I don't think I'm so unusual. [Cue sound effect of daughter sighing, 'Don't be so old fashioned. People simply don't operate like this anymore.'] Well maybe, but I know lots of women, most of them younger than I am, who all seem to want boyfriends that they can love and who will love them.

Then there are the married men who want to have 'uncomplicated' sex with single women without, of course, mentioning this to their wives. I never see how this can be good for them, for the single woman or for the wives. Is there any quality of sex that would be worth that level of heartache? I have done this, very briefly, and hated myself. Either everyone tells the truth to everyone and lets everyone deal with reality so that we can love each other as we are – or I'm not playing.

Another weird experience was being in a relationship with a man who wanted to have anal sex while I did not. Who wanted to try group sex while I did not. Who wanted ... well, he just wanted lots of things that I didn't, while I wanted a kind of emotional, mental and spiritual connection that he didn't seem to be interested in. I guess that's one definition of incompatibility – just being on totally different wavelengths, having a feeling that you are not really compatible and yet still trying and failing to make anything feel harmonious.

I've had lots of very bad sex.

• • •

So what else might women do on a tantric workshop? Eat delicious homemade curries? Sit by log fires? Maybe there will be stories about good sex? Now there is a subject women like to discuss with a glass of wine. But do I have any? There was a man once who lay in bed beside me and said, 'I'm shaking.' It wasn't cold but we were very much in love. I cherish that moment in my mind, heart, soul and body memory. We weren't even touching.

But back to the present. Sigh. The woman running the workshop is Hilly Spenceley, who I'd met once before, years ago when I did a mixed weekend that I wrote about in *The Battersea Park Road to Enlightenment*. Hilly. She's in her 70s: an earth mother archetype with a sense of humour. Having had six children by six different men (and now with an impressive 11 grandchildren) she's had a lot of experience of male sexual energy. Hilly has been a healer, a masseuse and a professional sex worker – a fact which she doesn't hide and says that, although it still shocks some people, the experience taught her a lot about men and sex. Hilly's been teaching tantric sexuality for 30 years. If we could clone people it would be a good idea to make millions of Hillys. Every town needs one, every village, every street.

I'm terrified of her. And somehow I'm about to overcome all my qualms and fears and go away with her and about thirty other women to some place that you'd never find on a map.

• • •

I always have a feeling of dread before any kind of retreat that requires work on the self, but the thought of an all-female workshop creates a silent inner scream. There is something about a group of women sitting in a circle that makes me think of witches. I have to become a witch. And I don't want to.

Resistance is all part of 'the process', apparently. The process is to change my perception of being a woman from 'female form of meat package that I just happen to have been born into but male would have been just as good, in fact considerably more useful in many ways,' to 'I am an incarnation of the Divine Feminine, the goddess Shakti, The Great Mother and I enjoy and celebrate that.' I swear if they could work growing more buxom breasts and giving birth to triplets into the timetable that would be included some time on Sunday morning.

I don't usually have negative feelings about being a woman (apart from immediately prior to workshops that is). But I don't have positive ones either. There is a famous prayer with which an orthodox Jewish male is encouraged to begin his day and it includes the line, 'Praised are You,

O Lord our God, King of the Universe, who has not made me a woman.' One curious prayer to be sure. But then I have never woken up feeling grateful that I am a woman either. Gender is something I've taken for granted rather than enjoyed. Perhaps women enjoy being women more when there are men around who enjoy them? Did our mothers and our grandmothers enjoy being women more or less than us, do you think?

My family has four generations of strong women on the maternal side. My great-grandmother, who I never met, had 13 children. My grandmother, Aimee, who raised me for the first six years of my life, lost her husband on my mother's 13th birthday and brought her four children up alone from that day onwards. My mother brought me up with no husband as she and my father separated before my birth. I was single as I raised my daughter.

In contemplating this heritage I have usually focused on the absence of men rather than the strength of the women. I'd love to have all four generations together at once – they would all be miraculously aged around 40 – to find out what they all think about being female. Can you imagine this conversation with your own mother, grandmother and great-grandmother? We'd have to go back quite a few more generations, I believe, before we found a woman who identified with the Mother Goddess. Maybe our ancestral mothers would all feel that having been female was more a curse than a blessing. If I'm honest, and I could choose between lifetimes (as some of the far out 'New Age' people believe that we can), I'd rather come back as a man. I've always felt a bit of a failure as a woman – as if I don't quite have what it takes. Which leads me right back to the purpose of the weekend. I've done so much spiritual work in which gender makes no difference that arriving on the tantric path is a shock.

Today's workshop has a most unpropitious beginning. To get to the unlocatable location you have first to go to Birmingham and then cast spells on taxi drivers who could not otherwise be lured so far from the safety of traffic jams. But this is no cavern with log fires. My fledging inner witch is mortified to arrive at a truly hideous residential centre featuring school-style dorms with plastic covers on the extra narrow bunk beds. Those running the workshop are apoplectic with apology, never having used this quick-build-take-the-money-and-run-before-it-falls-down venue before. They are 'smudging' the dorms by burning sage to disguise the smell of BO from whatever unfortunate lost beings were sleeping here last night. I glance at the other women attendees antagonistically wishing I could turn them all to stone with a glance. Can I go home now?

• • •

When we arrive in the main room after dinner I learn that they call their work a 'mystery school' so I can't tell you in detail about any of the particular processes that we are about to do. This doesn't prevent me from telling you what I experience; it just makes my job considerably harder and puts me into a worse mood. I mean obviously I want to tell you the spells. Dammit. The reason that they don't allow anyone to talk, specifically, about some of the methods is that half the women who come would never have the courage to show up if they knew what was going to be asked of them. Once here, miles from home and trapped in a silk web of encouragement from other women, breakthroughs are made. They want women to do this work and they don't want people like me misrepresenting it. This means that the only way I can tell you about all this is to consider the effect that it has on me. This is what I least want to do ... So I have to do the work with 100% integrity and then I hope that I can be of some help to you. Bleugh.

We are asked tonight to think about how we feel about being a woman at whatever age we are. I sit moodily and don't join in the conversation. Then they have a variation on this question about how we are feeling.

'How does your vagina feel?' This is just not the sort of question that gets asked every day. I say nothing but I think about it. I mean, physically or emotionally? Physically, right now, I can't feel it at all. I do not receive sensation from the vagina in the normal course of a day, or if I could then I'm unaware of it/her? How does it/she feel emotionally? A little confused at this point, I suppose. Certainly not confident. So it seems that today I have reflected that I'd be equally happy as a man and my vagina is dazed and confused.

We are now invited to consider our relationship with our breasts in a kind of meditation. They tell us that breasts nurture our children or our lovers, but we don't often think of nurturing our breasts or them nurturing us. I'm not speaking in terms of turning oneself on sexually, but just about nurture and gentle pleasure. It turns out that many women never stroke their own breasts. I agree – it's not a pastime that I've ever given a great deal of time to. 'How do we feel about our breasts?' There are the usual judgements, 'too big', 'too small', 'wrong shape'. And even if some women love them, don't we usually think of them as nurturing for babies or others? I've never considered mine as nurturing for me. Weird, witchy workshops.

In every 'process' we are invited to consider the wonder of the female body. I don't dislike mine but it's true I've taken it for granted. Even when it miraculously produced a child, I was young and I barely noticed the miracle. How can we enjoy being women or men more? These are not questions we usually consider in the normal working day. How many of us really celebrate the sex we are? I think of my friend who has waited 50 years to have a gender change and now, finally, is a woman. She wakes up every morning with amazed delight and joy to find herself in a female form.

• • •

We have been asked to bring objects that are sacred for us to place on the 'altar'. Someone has brought a statue of a Tibetan Buddhist, 'Shakti', and next to her is a 'Jewish Shakti'. Although it's not correct to call her that. She is Asherah, a copy of a statue from the Israel Museum. One of the participants has a special interest in the female depictions of the Divine in Judaism.

'She was once the consort of Yahweh,' she explains to me. 'Once there were female figures like her in every temple.'

'She is the goddess that Solomon would have had in his temple, but of course she was suppressed as Judaism became patriarchal.'

'And you don't often hear the Shekinah spoken of apart from in Jewish mysticism. That is the feminine in the presence of God. Hebrew has a word for this.'

This woman was beautiful. Somehow managing in herself to celebrate her femininity, her sexuality and her Jewish heritage – all in her own living form.

I must have been absent the week they covered sexuality in my confirmation classes in the Church of England.

'In Christianity I don't recall the feminine nature of God ever being spoken of. I'm very happy to see that you have brought your little Asherah statue to hang out with the girls in the 21st century.'

Someone else has brought the much-loved but widely misunderstood statue of Shiva having sex with his Shakti on his lap. This statue, although greatly admired for its apparent eroticism, is actually – in tantric cosmology – about the universe being perceived as being created, penetrated and sustained by the two forces which are in union: the masculine or abiding aspect of universal energy and the feminine or energetic aspect. People buy this statue of a rather beautiful copulating couple not realizing that it is actually about the nature of the character we have traditionally called 'God'. Anyway, they are here, the two of them, doing their thing.

And Ganesh is here, waving his long trunk about happily – quite why I didn't like to ask. 'He's a remover of obstacles,' someone tells me. Of course he is. You knew that didn't you? But does anyone actually pray to him? 'Please remove the competition, Ganesh?' As well as these more traditional offerings people have brought photos of their partners or yonic objects (that is, objects that resemble a yoni like a cowrie shell or the centre of an orchid flower).

The vulva, in the tantric tradition, is referred to as the 'yoni' – a Sanskrit term that takes a little getting used to. Some prefer 'pussy'. Please not the terms chosen by American teenagers: 'Junk' or 'goof'. At least let's have something affectionate. My daughter's friends choose 'Vajayjay', which sparkles and sounds like the female of 'vajra'.

On this course they do call the penis the 'vajra'. Vajra is a term that has so many different (but related) meanings that an entire page of Wikipedia is dedicated to it. But suffice to say that it often represents the male principle, or here – the penis. I assume the wit that has placed a banana on the altar is making a humorous reference to this revered and sacred item.

I have brought photos of my late grandmother, late mother and really quite punctual daughter in the hope that I can somehow do this work for all of us. My mother was elegant and graceful and my daughter has always seemed to be happier in her female incarnation than I am. Someone puts a large pink crystal phallus immediately in front of my mother's photo. They can't do this. It seems outrageous that she should have to look at it. Should I move it? Move my mother? Cover her eyes? I look at her photo and the huge erect penis. Were it not for a one-time proximity of these two forms I would still be in the ether waiting to be born but,

but, all the same ... I grasp the penis boldly and move it a good two feet away from her.

Why is it that we can never really imagine our parents having or enjoying sex? My daughter puts her fingers in her ears and sings, 'la la la la la' loudly if ever reminded where she came from or how she got in there so you can imagine her feelings on my writing this book.

'I'm traumatized, Mother. And I'm accepting voluntary contributions from readers toward my potential need for therapy.'

The thing is, your mother isn't supposed to do this sort of thing. You don't want to think about yours doing it either, do you?

I go on staring at my mother, realizing that maybe she'd have smiled at the oversized pastel pink crystal carving. Like all of our mothers, she must have had sex at least once.

At the top of the altar, in the centre, is an oil painting of a woman from the shoulders down. She has huge beautiful breasts and a rounded and large stomach or 'womb'. The 'womb' is described here as the seat of fertility, not just of babies but also of ideas, projects, nurture, everything. So this part of the body can still be enjoyed whether or not some of the older women have had their physical womb removed.

So I hope you now have a vision of the somewhat unconventional 'altar' that sits behind us as we work. There are pictures on my 'Sensation' Pinterest page if you'd like a look.[1]

After we've all looked at the altar, we sit on cushions and talk to each other. The introductions are always interesting.

Some are academics and some are women who have stayed home and brought up children. A policewoman, a barrister, a charity worker, a model – we are aged between 23 and 63. Some have been on the tantric path for 30 years and some started last night. In my estimation we are astounding just for being here.

We sit in our circle and discuss, for a while, all the subjects that really matter if we are to be fully ourselves. Birth, death and sex all happen behind closed doors. If you want to see a corpse to give yourself a reality wake-up call, unless the deceased is a family member it's almost impossible. The only way would be to feign an interest in becoming a professional embalmer and then, perhaps, with a lot of forms and permissions given, it would be possible to visit to remind yourself how you are going to look very soon. Birth is the same – unless you are fortunate enough to have a friend who invites you to be present at the birth of their baby or you have your child at home and invite others, it's unlikely that you will ever witness the birth of a child. And of course there is sex, we have all seen this, on television and online – versions so unlike what happens in most people's bedrooms that very little comparison can be made. How far most of us are from knowledge and daily awareness of our natural selves and our connection with all that lives and breathes.

Talking honestly about sex is hard. On Saturday morning I admit that I'd found the exercises on the previous night strangely threatening and even that I find being in a room with all these amazing women intimidating. Some women cry as they share their stories, admitting they want to run away or that they are not orgasmic or they just don't have a good time in bed with men in any way. But we have travelled here from all over the UK and some from other countries so, no matter how scared we are, no one is likely to run away. Recognizing ourselves in others, we want to keep the group complete and not allow any women to take her fears home with her. One woman has had a hysterectomy and feels that she has lost all her sexuality along with her womb. Two women are therapists but neither seem comfortable in their own skin. One woman admits that she had been married for 30 years and never had an orgasm. Several women say they have great sex and simply wanted to make their sex lives better still.

Inspiringly, one woman has been drawn here by seeing someone complete the tantra training and witnessed the transformation:

'She turned, metaphorically, into a beautiful red setter bounding out of the back of a car into the woods. That's the way she is now. The way that she is living her life.'

Three other women had come for that reason ... because they had seen the transformation in another woman.

And then there was me – as always trying to do the process fully and observe the process all at the same time. I'm supposed to be a bit stronger, older and wiser by now but I feel most like the younger women that just want to run away. But I'm also taking delight in being away for the weekend – far away from T, as if I had to claim my right to be a woman away with other women. Not that this right was ever taken from me, but women just don't do it. It feels as if, somewhere in our collective history, perhaps when we were all tribal, women would go away to the woods together to learn about sexuality, dance, sing and just celebrate being women. If women were ever to dance together, naked, as I did years ago on another seminar a bit like this one, they would soon see and learn that we are all different and that the idea, so prevalent today, that some body shapes are better than others, is utterly absurd. To be this natural and unselfconscious would be 'normal'. Crazy, isn't it?

The second morning there's a group of women in the showers all complimenting each other on how beautiful their breasts are. They're laughing and it's funny because some of the aforementioned breasts are huge and some are almost completely flat. Some have a huge areola and some barely any. We wonder how we've been brainwashed into believing that some shapes are better than others. We don't judge trees do we? 'Ah, look – that oak tree is better than that chestnut.' Or flowers: 'that daffodil is more attractive than that tulip.' How did we all become so judgemental? This simple act of comparison in which we assign labels 'better than' and 'worse than' has created several industries including, of course, the cosmetic surgery and the diet industry. When are we women going to just enjoy our bodies as nature intended and take care of them instead of so often destroying them with bad food, cigarettes and drugs?

Anyway, I'm just saying that I'm enjoying being with women now.

Hilly is very much the earth mother archetype. She helps women 'to be born into full realization of the beauty of their own bodies and the bliss available to them'. Quite a job. I once asked her about all the men in her life and the fathers of her children.

'When you were with father number six, did you sometimes find yourself wishing you were still with father number two?'

Hilly said, 'After a while I realized that they were all just different faces of the same God.' This is the best level. They are all 'Shiva', the masculine energy, just in different forms.

• • •

Whenever women meet together for this kind of work, you can guess that there will be some element of nakedness that you will be invited to experience. The process may sound corny or even dreadful to you. But if it does, then you're already joining in. Ask yourself why you would feel full of dread? Why would you not want to be seen naked by your sister women? Could you celebrate dancing naked just as a child would? Are you ashamed of your body? If so, on what grounds? If you are an older woman, have you failed in some way if you have a stomach that is not flat? If you are a younger woman, have you failed in some way if your breasts are not as large as another woman's? If you are a woman of 70 who has given birth to three children, have you failed if your body is not the same as it looked when you were 30? What exactly is there to be ashamed about? Don't just think 'I just wouldn't enjoy it.' If that is so, think about *why* you wouldn't enjoy it. And could you overcome that.

Any process, in any seminar, that involves nakedness

between women is utterly beautiful. Part of the tantric and sexual journey is about self-acceptance and we all need to learn what exactly we are not accepting and to acknowledge the insanity. It's always a surprise to learn that, no matter how beautiful a woman is, and how perfect her body is, she often remains focused on her own perceived inadequacies. Not just the most obvious 'my bum's too big' but beliefs that would really make you want to cry. A woman who has had children thinks her stretch marks are ugly? Or a woman with a beautifully perfect yoni thinks 'it's too big' or 'it sticks out too much'. Women – how did we become this insane? I imagine I can hear you wince if I use the word 'yoni', but even Eve Ensler who created *The Vagina Monologues* says that 'vagina' sounds medical. They call the vulva a yoni on this training, so yoni it is for now.

Why would nudity be scary? I've done lots of self-acceptance-type work over the years and, mostly, I feel pretty good about myself, but never having done any tantra, this work hasn't extended as far as my body so my absurd physical inhibitions have remained firmly intact. In my mind my breasts are too small, my stomach is too big, and even (how absurd is this?) my yoni is the wrong shape. Now please forgive me for mentioning this, and you may quite understandably feel that it really is too much information, but if I don't talk about these things then I am yet one more person playing into the taboo. So courage is called for. I know that the idea of one shape of yoni or vulva being potentially more attractive than another is absurd. I suppose I must have acquired this view from way back when I was a young teenager and saw my first porn magazine. I will have compared my own body to the bodies of the women that appeared there and naturally deduced that I was 'wrong' or 'weird'.

It's alarming that vaginal surgery, called 'labiaplasty', is one of the fastest growing areas of cosmetic surgery. And they don't even have to advertise. This isn't women who have anything wrong with their labial lips and they don't have surgery to improve sensation or pleasure, it can actually impede both. This is the cosmetic clipping of the folds of skin around the vulva. They want this because they, like the young teenage me, have seen the porn magazines where all the women have either been chosen because they have an unusually 'neat' shape (i.e. inner labial lips smaller than outer lips or barely visible at all), or because they have had themselves surgically altered for the cameras. The most requested surgery is called the 'Barbie' in which labia do not protrude at all. Thus we have another self-perpetuating industry. An irony is that in certain African cultures the inner labia are enlarged and even stretched because it has been noticed that larger inner lips increase the pleasure both for women and for men. In the West women want them chopped off.

How surgeons justify this I can't imagine. 'It's what she wants,' they will say to themselves I suppose. A little study on the tantric path could save women money and pain. I'm surprised a number of Harley Street practitioners haven't had Hilly's courses shut down as she is losing them business by teaching simple self-acceptance.[2]

•••

I've learnt to stand in my nakedness and to accept my body. I may still be some way from fully celebrating every part of it but I'm glad that I have a body that is healthy and, at the moment my feeling is, beautiful – at least to T. He tells me every day that he finds my various bumps and curves attractive. I can look at other women's bodies and see beauty. The shape of some women's breasts makes me want to rush to my life drawing class to draw them. I don't feel like this about my own body; but neither am I ashamed of it. I don't love it; but I don't dislike it either. So here I'm on a kind of middle ground between those who loathe their bodies and those who celebrate the skin they are in fully. Some women can't be naked. Can we really blame women's magazines? We have to take responsibility women – both for the way that we could enjoy and celebrate ourselves and for the sake of the men that want to love us.

Today, after a process that helped us to consider these things and drop some of the nonsense that we carry around, they played Shaina Noll singing 'How could anyone ever tell you that you're anything less than beautiful?'[3] If you'd like the soundtrack to this part of the workshop, you can download it yourself from iTunes for 99p. If you really want to understand the experience – take off your clothes sometime, look in the mirror and listen to Shaina's voice until you understand that you've somehow been brainwashed into seeing yourself as anything less than perfect, just as you are.

This may strike you as a little corny but if you choose to

take off your clothes in a room of strangers then the core of you that feels very vulnerable needs a little looking after, and if it helps – being sung to. Consider this please: male or female, we have all been influenced by the sales pitches that have to first convince us that there is something wrong with us so that they can profit by bringing us the solution. If necessary go the whole way, take your clothes off, stand in front of a mirror and play the song. Ask yourself – how did I ever get to imagine that I am less than perfect just as I am? If you are unhealthily over- or underweight that's a little different. It's good to drop extra weight to be as healthy as you can, and nourish your body sufficiently so it can move, dance and live. But even that doesn't imply that we aren't beautiful as we are ... just that we need to take notice if we are not looking after our health.

Today I saw a woman who was what doctors would call 'overweight' saying, 'I love the shape of my breasts; I love my stomach, which I associate with my daughter; I love my legs, they are strong and powerful; I love my arms, they are tender to hold, protect and nurture; I love my hair, it is thick and makes me feel feminine; I love my yoni, it gives me pleasure.' She was radiant and full of love for herself and for everyone around her. She is a woman who has completed this tantra training and is now back to assist other women. She dresses with celebration and is a joy to behold.

If more women felt like this about themselves how much happier this would make their men and how much better everyone's sex lives would be. One of the basics of a good sex life has to be how both partners feel about their own bodies. Sex is dependent on mutual enjoyment and how can a man really enjoy a woman's body if, every time he tells her that a part of her body is beautiful to him she replies, or even thinks, 'I don't agree.' And all this is, of course, true the other way around. How can a woman love a man who doesn't appreciate himself? How can she admire a man who doesn't admire himself? So we are back to the same message that the true journey is with ourselves. Don't you just hate that? Personal responsibility is so annoying.

Sometimes this work is surprising. This morning I was kissed in a very affectionate and loving way, on the forehead, by one of the other women. An older woman hasn't kissed me in that loving way since my mother was alive. And she died when I was 18 years old. Somehow I'd forgotten how tender older women can be. Very slowly I can feel the slight unnamed fear I had of working with a group of women melting away.

The final exercises of the day I can't tell you about specifically. The reason that this work is secret is not because there is anything sordid about it – quite the reverse, the work and all the processes are beautiful – but simply they are better experienced than written down on paper and because many would never pluck up the courage to do this work if they knew exactly what was going to happen.

So let's just say that if you've seen *The Vagina Monologues* you could probably take an imaginative guess at one of the processes. If you've not seen this play it involves performances from true-life recordings made of women who speak what their vaginas would say if they could talk.

The stories are profound and if, by any chance, you've not seen a performance of this award-winning piece of theatre, then I recommend you read the book – or listen to the yonis in the book. I have seen the performance on stage, twice, and while I enjoyed it very much and was impressed, each time, by the courage and conviction of the actresses – never did I stop to think of what my own vagina would say if given a voice. Of what stories she may tell.

But now I ask her I find she has a voice of her own and she says,

'I have been neglected, ignored, and never, never thanked. You have called me ugly, accused me of not being the right shape. You have told me that I don't perform the way you like. Although I delivered for you a perfect daughter you have never valued, appreciated, treasured or loved me. T loves me. How is it that he feels more positive about me than you do yourself? He adores me but you are indifferent to me. He wants to be close to me but you don't care for me. I would like to be enjoyed, not only by T but by you. And I'd like to be drawn.'

'What?' I say in alarm. 'You're kidding me. You're not the prettiest thing in the world you know.'

Silence.

'I'm sorry. I didn't say that you were ugly. I just didn't realize that you could possibly want a portrait.'

'To be drawn you have to really look, and you have to let yourself be seen. Ask T if you don't want to do it. He'd like to draw me I'm sure.'

'You're right. I think he may be more keen than I am.'

No one can say I'm not broadminded. I'm having a conversation with my own vulva and letting you listen. Before you condemn me as weird, listen to *The Vagina Monologues*. Then listen to your own, if you have one – give her a voice and let her talk to you. Well, you thought this book may contain some weird challenges, I guess? If you have a penis you may be well aware of what he has to say to you. And even though a man's relationship with his penis can sometimes be a complex and troubled one, few men forget them. Many have even given their penis a name. I've a friend who calls his 'Justin'. He always knows what Justin has to say.

• • •

By the last day of the workshop I was surprised, as I always am, by the grace and sheer magnificence of my fellow women. If you give women a process – a challenge that is difficult – most women will run at it with courage, almost with wings. We humans are inspirational. Give us a chance and most of us want to move beyond our limitations. Both women and men want to be happy and enjoy our lives to the full. Sometimes when we 'settle' for unhappy lives, it's only because we lack the tools and the know-how to dig out a path to something better. This is what these workshops do. This is what all human potential work does. And while so many in the intelligentsia and the most literate and erudite mock the 'self-help' section of the book store ... those who read those books are gently helping themselves to ways out of problems, to thinking in new ways and creating better lives.

When you give people the tools, as Hilly is doing here with us this weekend, people will build better lives for themselves.

I'm not saying human potential work is easy or that transformation can be achieved in a weekend. But a kind of thawing can begin, a new openness. Women will go away and read some more books, be more attentive to themselves, maybe buy a new dress, throw away some of the old knickers and buy something more beautiful. As these women return to their homes their husbands or partners may notice more light in the eyes, a slightly different posture that is not so apologetic, even a subtle new eagerness between the sheets.

The next course that I will be doing is much more fun. It's a couples' weekend. T is full of enthusiastic anticipation.

Tantric Sex Workshop for Couples

In the café where I'm writing this I've just asked six men a simple question: 'Who do you think is more interested in sex – men or women?' Five answer 'men', one answers 'women'. Now that is hardly a large sample of the population but I think their answers reflect the established view that men are more interested in all forms of sex. What is it that we are told by the popular magazines? That men think about sex every seven seconds?

T arrives. 'It's not true at all. I just rode over here on my bike. It was a 25-minute bike ride and I only thought about sex four times.'

'Thank you for that clarification.' Sigh.

Women, we are told, rarely think about it at all. During sex we are apparently thinking about shopping or that the ceiling needs painting. Maybe women really do think about sex less often. But this doesn't mean that women are less interested in sex. If you change the focus from regularity of sexual thoughts to a desire for quality in sexual experience, then the answer is reversed. The men, it seems, think about sex more and want sex more often. The women want quality; they want better sex.

On the couples' tantra trainings it is always the women who have dragged the men along – sometimes kicking and screaming. For a man to come to any weekend with the words 'sex' and 'training' in the same workshop description – he has to be willing to be open to the radical concept that he may have something to learn. For T this is not a problem simply because he is interested in anything and everything that will lead to any variation on 'more sex'.

'What man wouldn't want to learn a million ways to please a woman and be pleased by her?' he asks.

'Sadly, many men.' I tell him.

So here we are. Away in the countryside on a weekend called 'An Invitation to Pleasure – Level One: Desire.' We are one of six couples and there is the usual range of ages and backgrounds. We have a large private room with a comfortable double bed and a view of fields. The birds are singing outside and I'm singing inside. I'm in a good mood this time. We have a couple running the group. For me it's very reassuring to have men around. They are our brothers after all and I like the feeling of us learning together.

Sometimes there are women in the women's workshops who have had a bad time with men and there can be a feeling of women discovering their sexuality in spite of men. Personally I prefer all of us discovering our strengths, vulnerabilities and weaknesses together.

I enjoy the range of couples here too. One couple includes a pregnant woman. They have been together some years and are here to enrich the sexual area of their lives at a time when many couples are struggling with it. And she wants to find out how to continue to feel sexy through her pregnancy and as a young mother. They are so loveable I want to wrap them in ribbon and grant all their wishes forever.

There is an older couple. The woman has done all the women's workshops and has now brought her terrified husband along. Bless him. There is a pair of young partners who have done every kind of training and have thrown away anything that could be remotely called an inhibition. They are impressive and the rest of us are rather in awe of them. Then there are two other couples, each touching in their own way. And then T and me. I am happy/terrified/excited and T looks like the tomcat who got the cream.

A couples' workshop is a lot gentler than the women's work. The couple running it, Sue Newsome and her partner Martin Hellawell, look very down to earth compared to some of the mystical-looking teachers you sometimes find running workshops of this kind. She describes herself as a 'short Northerner in her 50s' and Martin is a 'tall Southerner in his 60s'. They are not the least intimidating, which is a good thing as they explain that you have to take things slower with men. You remember the word 'gentlemen'? Ladies and gentle men? And they are, so often, gentle. Anything that involves talking about sex instead of just getting on with it and they are often more scared than women are. So we start gently.

The first night we consider different ways of being together and apart. Again, it's such a myth, the idea that men tolerate women's need for love so that they can have sex and women tolerate the sex so that they can have love. It's all so much more subtle and complex than that.

There are many drives to the sexual act. One of them is instinctive biological desire to have sex because it feels good. But there are others. A desire to feel connected? An admiration of someone that is so intense that you just want to rip your clothes off and get as close to them as you possibly can? A co-dependent desire to please the other to win approval? A need for reassurance? A quick and easy cure for your insomnia? A need to get out of the brain and into the body? A desire to have triplets with this person? A list like this could be long. As a starter for our weekend we considered, with various exercises, different ways of being together and apart. I love these processes. There is a memorable passage in Kahlil Gibran's *The Prophet*, which is sometimes read at weddings, where Gibran writes, in answer to the question 'Speak to us of marriage', about the fact that two trees must not lean on each other nor grow, one in the shade of the other but instead each must grow alone with the other beside them. Each with their roots in the earth and their leaves in the sun.

I'm not sure that Sue and Martin could teach us all everything we need to know about co-dependency and fully functional interdependence in one evening, but to maximize the chance of relationships working we could at least cover the basics. I have always loved the discussion of what makes relationships successful. I kept reaching for my notebook to write down the wisdom in précis.

'There need be no drama if our partner can't meet our desires or requests.'

'I do not need his/her approval.'

'The less attached you are, the more likely you are to get what you want.'

'You can be a king and a queen in your relationship. Neither of you need be a beggar.'

'Please use dental floss.'

No – they didn't really mention dental floss. They missed an opportunity there to save many a couple from the divorce courts, I thought.

I also thought we needed to stop and spend at least a day discussing each of those ideas. How can we base our relationships less on need and more on choice? This, in short, is what makes so many relationships unhappy. They are leaning on each other like Gibran's first two trees. Sometimes this can work to an extent but more often it leads to feelings of resentment. If a couple have both learnt to live happily alone and instead are choosing to live together – the relationship is not one of dependency but one of choice.

Sadly, our current society is so obsessed with what psychologists call 'the romantic myth' that there are increasingly fewer of us that have ever lived alone. I blame Hollywood. There are relationships where the couple feel unable to be apart – ever. There are adults that have never been to the cinema alone or eaten in a restaurant alone and can't even endure the sound of the thoughts inside their own heads. Yet we expect others to live with us. And call this love. Ha ha ha.

Sue and Martin have one evening to explore this with us. Can we thrive and be joyful whether together or apart? There is one simple exercise where we move together and apart across the room. I end up not being sure whether it's good or bad that I prefer looking at T from across the room. Come in, Dr Freud. But I love the feeling of wanting to walk toward him. Especially when he has the sense not to walk toward me so that I have to move if I want to be closer to him. The most profound learning can come from these simple games.

Years ago a Tai Chi teacher whom I was rather taken with told me off for always wanting to be close to him. 'How can I move toward you,' he asked, 'if you are always moving toward me? There are natural laws – action, re-action; pull, push. You will never experience me wanting to come toward you if you don't give me space and distance.' And it was true – I always wanted to be right by his side. So I learnt this one. It was fun, now, to explore it with T in a literal way by us moving toward and away from each other in physical space.

You'll know this one if you've ever been in a relationship where the person always wants to be close to you. I remember a brief relationship years ago where I would end up clinging on to the edge of the bed. The phrase, 'Darling, please will you give me a little space?' ceased to be metaphorical. It went on all day and all night until, inevitably I suppose, I did push him away.

So T and I are here learning how to avoid this one – I hope. When he moves toward me I want to walk backwards, away from him, to preserve the space but if he stands still then I want to move toward him. This, on this day, is the dynamic between us and everyone around us has a different dynamic. 'Why do you always do that?' one partner asks another when the discussion about the exercise happens afterwards.

'Do what?'

'Move away when I move toward you?'

'You move too fast,' said the woman, daring to be honest.

'Oh,' said the man. 'I get it'

What is sometimes called 'The Dance of Intimacy' is clearer when you see it played out literally like this. It's often easier for us to want someone we don't have, than someone we do. And how does this obvious fact tip over into the dynamics of longing and desire in sexuality? Discuss? With your beloved one night?

Then we have another simple process, more about relationship than sexuality, in which we are asked to consider three things that we appreciated about each other when we first met and three things that we appreciate now.

It's good to hear what we are bringing to a relationship and what is most enjoyed. Our power to be a positive influence on ourselves is limitless. This, then, takes all the pressure off your partner. If we concentrate on fixing ourselves then we'll have no energy left to be critical of the other and, ideally, can just enjoy receiving feedback on how we are doing. It takes two playing fairly though to make this work.

Any lover that gives their partner unsolicited 'feedback' on where the other is going wrong deserves a death stare and some kind of punishment that doesn't involve delight or chocolate.

We ended the night by exploring energy through 'melting hugs' – a kind of full body hug (no pelvic thrusting) where you simply enjoy the energy of the other person. Do you ever wonder what exactly people are bathing in when they bathe in your energy? Jill Bolte Taylor (of the best-ever TED talk. Watch it later...[4]) asks us to be responsible for whatever energy we bring to a space. If only it were as easy to be as aware of our own energy as it is to be of other people's.

That night T dreams that he saves me from a huge bunch of men. He says to me in the morning in a half-awake state, 'You came to me but then I let you go. You let me go free.' Listening to him I smile. He's not sure whether I let go of him or he let go of me.

• • •

Our Saturday morning exercises and discussions are about saying 'no'. It's very important to be able to say this simple word before anyone can really say 'yes' to anything.

'Would you like to watch cheap porn in bed tonight before we have sex?'

'No thanks.'

'Would you like to be tied up, denigrated and humiliated?'

'Er – not on Thursdays, thanks.'

'Would you like to do something involving faeces?'

'No, thanks. I don't indulge before breakfast.'

It's good for us, the women especially it seems, to establish what they call 'an authentic "no"'. This is very hard for some women and plays a part in my own journey. My first husband arrived in the relationship with me from a relationship where a previous woman had apparently rejected him for many years. With the wisdom and maturity you would expect from a girl in her early 20s I decided that I would never reject him and, for the seven years that I was with him, I never did. As I had not attended one of these workshops, no older and wiser woman had ever explained to me that if I never said 'no' then I could never say 'yes'.

'How many of you find it hard to say "no"?' All the women's hands go up. The men admit genuine surprise. They don't seem to understand why women lie to them.

It seems that the younger me isn't alone. Women don't like the men that they love to feel rejected. Most women are very good at empathy and know how rejection feels and they want to make the men that they are with feel happy and satisfied. 'I've got a headache' has become a cliché because the man knows that it's not necessarily honest. What she actually means is, 'I don't want to have sex with you tonight.' But if she says that, this begs the question, 'Why not?' Maybe what she is experiencing is not so pleasurable? But as she may not want to address that her excuses become more numerous.

This is an example of women (and I am certainly guilty of this) being cowardly and not doing what needs to be done for us to create better sex lives for ourselves. This, in turn, is disempowering for men as an honest 'no' gives them the compliment of assuming that they can deal with the rejection. And if they can't, it gives them the opportunity to learn how. In a relationship that is aiming at improving and deepening, it can lead to an honest conversation about why it's a 'no'. But we are never taught these things because few people do workshops like this one.

A woman says, 'Every time he is sexually aroused I feel responsible for him having pleasure from that.'

Women often feel that an erect penis is a 'job' for her whether she feels like it or not. I remember a man saying to me, 'Look at that!' as if his erection were my issue or his gift. Now I'm braver I'm able to say, 'I salute you. Please stand down.'

Sue and Martin tell the women very clearly that what's important is that she is 'in choice'. Many women are not choosing 'no' because they want the man's approval.

I wonder just how common this is so the next friend that phones me – I ask her.

'I'm terrible at saying "no". And I'm always aware of the repercussions. That isn't to say I don't from time to time, but it's a judgement call.'

'What are the repercussions?'

'Lots actually. He may be less willing to make the effort for me if he is tired and I am not. I'll have to live with him not having relieved his stress. He's less likely to sleep well and I don't want to reject because I don't like feeling rejected.'

She has four children. Oh, please! Men, it's really

important to realize that if you had a body that has energetic rhythms and cycles that are not constant but go up and down and then you have children making demands on you from the moment you wake up until the moment you collapse into bed you may find that you desire nothing more than sleep.

A woman lying next to a man with an erection can experience it as a desirable offering of love and pleasure or as yet another demand or need. This is why it is so important for a woman to be able to say 'no' when she wants to. So that the man knows that when she says 'yes', it's a real, 'Yes, please.'

You may all have one possible solution to this dynamic: 'Just take yourself in hand, man.' But I'm just relaying all this so that you know that it's not always as simple as the dynamic that one friend describes within his marriage:

Him: 'Yeah?'

Her: 'Nah.'

Him: 'Kay.'

This husband says he's fine with this because on other occasions she'll say, 'Yeah.' One girlfriend writes, 'I find that fake snoring and dribbling usually does the trick.' When I posed this question online, a man writes to me saying that no woman has ever said 'no' to him. I worry about him. Doesn't he realize that this isn't something he should be boasting about?

Can we aim at something better and more honest than the fake dribbling? Can we have relationships where neither approaches the other as a beggar? Where we can each ask for what we'd like clearly, confidently and without feeling as if we are begging?

Sue and Martin speak to us about being kings and queens in our relationships.

'If you are a queen, you do not beg from a king. If you are a king, you do not beg from the queen. It is possible to feel, both of you, as if you have everything that you need for you both to feel bountiful. An experience of bountiful abundance is what we are aiming at.'

Isn't 'abundance' a wonderful word?

How unexpected that to become a queen, we women need to start with 'an authentic "no"'. So simple for some and so hard for others.

• • •

They teach us a little about breathing. There are classic exercises that are described in Margo Anand's book *The Art of Sexual Ecstasy* that I have never made time to explore. I start to study this book when I get home and instantly go into overwhelm. In theory I should know about all the chakras and the role that they play in sexuality and I should know how, using breathing, to open my inner flute. At this point I go and make a coffee and complain to my houseguest, Jovanna, who is wiser than I am. Being American and from the West Coast, she has done everything. Naturally.

'What on earth is an inner flute? I'm sure mine is closed and should be open. How do I open it? There must be lots of people out there having great sex that have never even heard of an inner flute?'

She smiled sagely. 'Actually Isabel, I'm not sure that

there are so many people out there having great sex. Don't worry about the inner flute ... but you have tried the jade egg, haven't you?'

I drank my coffee.

'No, Jovanna. What's a jade egg?'

'It's a sacred practice that I experienced in South Africa.'

'Yeeesssss.'

'To increase the orgasm.'

I waited.

'I have a jade egg.'

'How big is this egg?'

'It's the size of an egg.'

'Thanks for that.'

'A well-fed chicken's egg.'

'You put the tip on your yoni. The yoni says "yes" or "no."'

I sipped my coffee. Does everyone have guests like this?

'If the yoni says "no" you stop. If the yoni says "yes" the yoni eats the egg and it gets sucked into the abyss.' She laughed. 'I've actually done this.'

'And the point of this is what?'

'To strengthen the pelvic floor muscles which are the muscles that you have to use to hold the egg in place.'

'Yes ...'

'But then you are moving it inside and you are very focused and it moves around and, I think, stimulates the G-spot, and after about 20 minutes I had the best orgasm I've ever experienced.'

'You had an orgasm from your yoni eating a jade egg?'

'I did. In a workshop. A bit like the workshops you've

been doing. Only different. Anyway, the problem came when I went home and tried to re-create the experience. I bought the book to practise at home.[5] In the book she has you boil the egg first to avoid infection, but the egg can't touch the bottom of the pan because it will crack. I had to take dental floss and tie it to the egg to stop it touching the bottom. There is a frustratingly tiny hole through the middle of the egg that's almost impossible to get the floss through – especially as I was getting very worked up. Then I boiled the egg and then of course it has to cool to the right temperature to avoid major yoni scarring. But my excitement was peaking to re-create my African experience. I decided to follow the instructions and start the first exercise standing.'

'And your yoni liked having a jade egg pushed into it?'

'No. I experienced huge disappointment as my yoni said a clear "no" and the egg went clattering to the ground onto the wooden floor. Rolling on the floor rather defeated the purpose of the boiling but by this time I didn't care and just rinsed it as I was in such a hurry to try again. After several attempts, the egg banging on the floor and an increasing fear that the neighbours would think I was knocking, I decided to lie down. I was quite excited that the yoni now said "yes" and once again sucked the, now fortunately cooled-off, egg into the abyss.'

My yoni was relieved to hear that her egg had cooled.

'Sadly I had not cut the floss long enough and found myself fishing in the abyss for the floss.'

'Seriously?'

'Yes, really. You're supposed to cut the floss long. So after what seemed like hours of no orgasmic experience whatever – and instead, me getting increasingly agitated at not being able to find the floss or remove the egg – I gave up.'

'But surely if you had just stood up, gravity would have helped you lay the egg?'

'No. Once it's in, it's in. You'd better make sure that you have a string long enough to fish it out.'

'So, what did you do?'

'I drank a few glasses of wine, went back to fishing and eventually located it.'

'Thank God. I thought you were going to say that you had to take yourself to hospital to find a long-fingered gynaecologist. So was that the end of the jade egg?'

'No. You'll be reassured, no doubt, to know that I've since then had several further more successful egg sessions. With longer floss.'

'And orgasm?'

'Oh, yes. But the egg is really for exercising the pelvic floor muscles. They recommend other exercises to strengthen the G-spot muscle.'

'The G-spot is a muscle?'

'I think so. Isn't it?'

'No – it's erectile tissue, surely? Or just an area where a lot of women have a collection of nerve endings? The same collection of nerve endings as the clitoris.'

'I think you're right. Hold on.'

She consulted the world wide web of sexual knowledge.

'On netdoctor.com they seem confused about whether the G-spot exists or not. They quote research here that says that in 1981 one woman experienced a stronger orgasm when the frontal wall of her vagina was stimulated and they called it the G-spot in honour of Gräfenberg, the author of a study in 1944. In 2001 scientists declared it a myth. In January 2010 a team from King's College London also declared that it didn't exist but their research was later found to be weak. The next year a group of French scientists declared that 56% of women have a G-spot.'

'Oh great. So we may not have one at all then? And there is my poor boyfriend trying to stimulate a spot I may not have or may not be important. No wonder I'm confused.'

'But can you feel it?'

'Well, I can feel more sensation from some areas than others but whether it's the G-spot I'm feeling or not I really don't know.'

'It says here that some women say that they definitely have one. Some say they definitely don't. Some say that stimulating it is wonderful, some say it just feels uncomfortable and some say only that it makes them want to pee.'

This is absurd. We can put men on the moon but we don't know even this much about pleasure in our own bodies? I may have to have another coffee.

'It also says here that a woman would have a hard time finding her own G-spot unless she has very long fingers. It also says that it can only be stimulated with the penis if you are sitting astride him and then leaning right back.'

I stopped to check all this. Enough theory and academic debate. There is a woman who has a career teaching about G-spots. I'm not going to do one of her seminars. But if you want to explore she's called Deborah Sundahl.[6]

'OK, Jovanna – I'll try all the weird positions in the *Kama Sutra* that I'm flexible enough to get into. Now stop talking to me about jade eggs. I'm telling the story of my weekend workshop with T and how wonderful it was.'

'But you can't write much specifically about what you actually did right?'

'It is a problem. I have to leave out some of the best bits.'

She laughed. 'OK, well you do that and I'm going to read about penises. It says here that self-measurement of the penis is notoriously unreliable.'

'Stop Jovanna. I'm trying to write here.'

'And results tend to be skewed by men who falsely claim to be 10 or 11 inches long.'

'I'm writing about my workshop. I was just saying that we had introductions to the chakras and the inner flute and that, as introductions, they served me well to teach me just how little I know. Do you think your chakras are open?'

She laughed. 'Forget my chakras – I'd like to get my legs open.'

'I was attempting a serious question. Which of your chakras do you think are open and which are closed?'

'What's a chakra anyway?'

'According to *The Art of Sexual Ecstasy*, the chakras are "symbolic representations of the energy fields created by the body's endocrine system".'

I have a picture of them on my Pinterest page, of the body with all these points in different colours ...[7]

'So, if you believe that you have them, which of your

chakras are open – do you think?'

'Jovanna?'

'My root chakra is definitely open, I cracked it open with a jade egg. The next one up my son kicked open trying to bust out. My heart chakra was busted open by a few bastards. My throat chakra – let's see ...'

'Jovanna, your throat chakra is open. You have no problem with communication.'

'My crown chakra is now shut down. It used to be open but then I started thinking more about sexuality and it got completely confused and shut down.'

'You've missed one.'

'I have?'

'The third eye. Intuition.'

'Ah yes – I forgot it. That's shut down too. I've read too much.'

'OK,' I said. 'I'm convinced that only my heart chakra is totally open. Yes, like you, a man opened mine, walked in years ago and then left it open as wide as a barn door. It's very painful having a heart chakra wide open. I feel everyone, everything. People talk about us all being "One" as if it's just a concept. But I feel it. It's very inconvenient. First I couldn't eat cows, then pigs, then chickens, and then fish. My love extends to rats and snails and slugs – now I have problems killing a mosquito. I apologize before pulling up a lettuce. I feel life in rocks. Thank God that all my other chakras are closed if this is the result of having just this one open.'

'I think all your chakras are open.'

'Thank you, Jovanna – that's very reassuring.'

• • •

Back to the workshop and the use of words. Whoosh. Cross-cut from my home to couples sitting in a circle in floppy clothes. We had thought about 'no'. The next words that we explore are 'yes' and 'wait'. Both are equally difficult words for some of us to express in a sexual context. I remember having a discussion with a woman once when I was giving her a shoulder massage and she was giving me zero feedback. I said to her, 'Hello? I need feedback – you know, words like, "yes", "no", "harder", "softer", "up a bit", "push harder right there".'

'I don't give feedback,' she said. 'Can't you feel what needs to be done?'

'Well, to an extent I can. But it really helps if you also give me guidance. Don't you give your husband feedback – on shoulder massage or during sex?'

'No. I expect him to be able to feel and know.'

She actually said that. Really. Ah, women – the myth of the man who understands us instinctively. Maybe they exist in fiction? Or after a lot of training in sexuality, which very few men get – or, well ... how many in a hundred really understand instinctively? Most of us don't understand ourselves, so I'm not sure we can expect a man to.

'Let's practise,' I ventured radically. 'Do you prefer it if I press the knots in your shoulder muscles harder or softer?'

I sound confident, don't I? Well, I'm fine at giving feedback with shoulder massage but curiously quiet with 'yes', 'no' or 'wait' in bed. Here it was great to practise with games. T hates being tickled. If I touch him anywhere on the sides of his body I know I'm going to get a loud 'no!' out of him. So I blew raspberries on his side to make it easy. And as for the word 'wait' – well obviously, I could write a chapter about that word. A huge amount of everything that goes wrong in much lovemaking comes from women's inability to say 'wait'. So gently, gently, we are here practising. And laughing a lot.

• • •

Jovanna interrupts again. (How am I supposed to get on with the narrative with a guest like this?)

'Did you do female ejaculation on the course?'

'No. They do courses for that?'

'Yes, you should talk to my friend Sabine. She did a workshop in Germany where a group of women learnt to ejaculate. I think they helped each other. Most of the workshops in Germany, as far as I can work out, seem to be groups of women stroking each other's clitoris and G-spot and having a lot more success than the men do.'

'But I'm straight.'

'So's Sabine.'

Do-it-yourself squirting with the help of other women? This is a workshop I will not be exploring. No publisher could pay me enough. If anyone writes to me and says, 'I went to Germany and did a women's "How to Squirt" workshop,' I'll buy any reader that does this a coffee on Battersea Park Road.

Back to the couples' workshop, the kind of work I'm assuming some of you may be open to exploring. We were in the late Saturday afternoon by now and moving into the evening. Many of the processes had been, in one way or another, about giving up control or taking the lead. Take a simple game (and you can play this at home) called 'One Hour, One Hour' – you can play with a lover, a mother, a friend or a child. You need a day ideally or just an afternoon.

What you do is that you take turns choosing what you are both going to do for the next hour. It's that simple. And huge fun. All you need is a willingness to take complete responsibility for the experience that you both have for an hour and then you also need to be flexible enough to do anything the partner chooses. This is very different from the way some couples normally operate by negotiation.

'Would you like to go to the cinema, dear? Or out for a meal?'

'Oh, I don't know. You decide.'

'Really, whatever you'd like.'

'I'm easy really – you choose.'

And so on until you lose the will to live. Or do what the other person chooses, have a bad evening and then get cross with them for making a bad choice and yourself for not having chosen.

Instead it can work like this. Flip a coin – you win. So you decide you'd like to spend the first hour with your playmate making you both breakfast while you read a book in bed. Your playmate then chooses the next hour, let's say they choose to go for a bike ride so at the end of the second hour you're on the other side of the park. Then you might say, 'OK, I'd like to go around this art gallery.' Then an hour later the choice may be, 'OK, now I'd like to cycle to this great pub on the river for lunch.' And so on. This game is wonderful for children who are not used to being able to choose the activities that 'grown-ups' do. And it can also be played with whole families taking turns. On holiday with my daughter we'd play 'One Day, One Day'. It avoided arguments fantastically. On my days we'd wake up at 5am, take a local bus and go sightseeing and have culture days. On her days we'd lie in and stay on the beach. She was forced to admit that it worked well. On my days I'd say, 'Let's walk down this street and explore,' and if she said, 'Why?' I'd say, 'Because it's my day and I'm curious.' And as she had agreed to play, that was the end of it.

I once played this with a child of four and had huge fun doing finger painting and playing ball and taking a bus just for the fun of it. In my hour, I had chalks and we went and drew pictures on the pavement.

And once I played with a boyfriend. It's particularly fun in bed.

This was the aspect that we were exploring in the couples' workshop. First there is the element of giving up control and then there is the element of asking for what you want for an hour. Of course there are boundaries and this is perhaps why we started the day with finding 'an authentic "no."' For example, ... anal (and please forgive me for speaking so frankly but this is a book about sex after all). Anal sex has never been my thing – so if T had started the evening saying, 'I'd like an hour's anal sex please,' then I'd have said 'no'. As it was I got lucky and it was my turn to start. I said,

'I'd like an hour's massage please – here's the oil.' I took off nearly all my clothes and lay face down in our little corner. Everyone else was doing whatever they wanted so no one was paying much attention to anyone else. Now of course T and I enjoy massaging each other normally, as many couples do, but we rarely dedicate an hour to it and if we do it's usually reciprocated. Here I had asked for an hour after only one day's practice of asking for what I want and only brief rehearsal of saying 'yes' and 'no'.

'What did you do on Saturday evening?' interrupted my houseguest again.

'Well, we continued that exercise until we went to bed.'

'And were people, you know, brave in their choices?'

'Some were. Some weren't.'

'And were you allowed to leave the main room?'

'Yes. Some left, some stayed. It was really beautiful actually. The room kind of felt like a mystical womb of some kind, dark and velvety. Each couple's nest was made up with beautiful silks and cushions. It felt very honouring with couples learning how to love and please each other.'

'Do they do this stuff for singles?'

'Yes. They have workshops just for women and they have mixed workshops.'

'You're not going to tell me about Saturday night then?'

'No. But I'll say that T is more OK with asking for what he wants than I am. I enjoyed his choices more than I enjoyed my own.'

Having told you that I'm not allowed to describe the processes that we do in these workshops because then everyone would be too frightened to attend – neither do I want your imaginations to run away with you. So yes, we had a lot of fun taking turns with an 'ask for what you want' process. But, well, let's just say that we were only playing with our own partners and not with anyone else's – and that the room was dimly lit.

As I write the final sentence about the Saturday – a voice comes from the corner of my lounge.

'Can I tell you more about jade eggs now then?'

'No. I'm going to bed.'

• • •

'Good morning, Jovanna.' I say the following morning, rubbing my eyes and pouring tea.

'So you've never tried a jade egg, Isabel? You haven't?'

'No, I once bought what they call "love eggs" from Ann Summers and they were so painful after I'd – what was the phrase you used – "launched them into the abyss" that I gave them exactly two chances before deciding that "the yoni said 'no'". In fact, my yoni said "no thank you" really very clearly. Let me show you.' I found my 'love eggs.'

'This looks like a dog toy.'

'Forget what it looks like – surely it serves the same purpose? But when I put these strange objects inside me, unsurprisingly they just hurt.'

'We have pleasure, pain or paralysis. So pain is good.'

'Why?'

'Paralysis is bad. Would you rather have a sore leg or a numb leg? Believe me – pain is good. But don't put those inside you because they look like a dog toy. At this stage in my life nothing is going in my yoni unless it looks good. The jade eggs are the Fabergé eggs of the sex world. But listen – I'm single. I've got to get creative.'

Commercial Break. 'Single? Forget looking out for a man to be your playmate, lover and friend – get yourself an exquisite jade egg! Simpler to operate than a man with none of those unexpected extra expenses. Jade eggs come in varying sizes so you can find the perfect egg for you.'[8]

No, I'm not on commission. Now where was I? Sunday morning of the workshop. The breakfast was great.

'There was a process we did on touching,' I told Jovanna. 'It was wonderful. My arms haven't been touched or kissed as well since.'

'Did you do touching with a feather?'

'We might have done.'

'Oh, I love that. I did a process like that once in South Africa and we took hours just touching very lightly. It was sheer heaven.'

I can reveal that since the couples' workshop T and I have been and purchased, from a posh sex shop, a very long black feather on a stick. It's a genuine thing of beauty. And I do enjoy asking to be stroked with it, ever so gently, for extended periods of time. And so does he. It's lovely if you are really tired and have time but no energy.

'Isn't it weird that slow, light touch has to be taught?' Jovanna said, sipping her tea.

'I guess it goes against our "more, stronger, harder, faster" culture. There was a point I remember when T was moving his finger down my arm so slowly that it was barely perceptible – and even then it felt too fast.'

'Yes, and with a feather you can barely feel it and yet it brings all your senses alive.'

Please make sure you are visualizing a peacock feather. Long, wispy and beautiful.

We all discussed what we had learnt from the previous day. Especially from the Saturday evening. I admitted that I had enjoyed T's choices more than my own. I love the fact that although in some areas of our lives I am much more confident than T is – around sexuality it is always T who takes the greater risks. Yet he's also patient with me.

We had one more technical exercise. Breathing is another subject, like the chakras, which seems to be key to everything. On Sunday there was an introduction to 'The Mirror Breath' and how this can be linked with pelvic rocking. I guess that eventually this exercise can be done naked and plugged in, so to speak ... but today I was having trouble even getting the breathing right.

'There was no obligatory nakedness?' Jovanna asked again.

'No, Jovanna. The whole course is an invitation so you can do just as little or as much as you want. But, just as with a body massage, it's difficult to do some things with your clothes on. Anyway, what's wrong with nakedness?'

'God, I really wouldn't want to take off my clothes even in front of women ... let alone if there were men in the room.'

'We were working with our own partners and concentrating on them. We were not ogling other people's partners. It was really a very safe and loving space that they created, and even the older man who came who was unaccustomed to any work of this kind was comfortable with the work we did. The women's work is much harder.'

'I find working with women easier.'

'I don't.'

'Why not?'

'Something genetic in me, Jovanna.'

'OK ... Anyway ... I've got to go now. I'll leave you to your writing. Do you like writing?'

'I do, yes. I'm talking to two people now about all this, you and the one reading. I try and hide nothing from the one reading. So it's hard for me that I'm not allowed to talk about everything that happens in these workshops ... and I try to imagine the questions. Anyway let me get on with my story.'

• • •

So, where was I? Sunday, last process. At the end of the weekend the processes moved away from sex and came back to love. It's amazing what we can be for each other in a relationship if we know how. A good woman can be playmate, mother (in a good way), child, lover, friend, goddess (in a good way), whore (in a good way), teacher, pupil, soulmate, guide and loving companion. A good man can be a woman's best friend, playmate, lover, teacher, pupil, father (in a good way), son (in a good way), protector and loving companion. And these are only some of the roles that we can play for each other.

So in our last process we explored this and ended up holding each other like children, each couple in our own little nest. Sue and Martin played beautiful music and looked at us all. And cried.

I know many celibates – I have more than an average number of nuns and monks of different traditions in my address book – who live and thrive without sex. When there is a choice to live without sex in order to pursue an exclusively spiritual life within a tradition, the nuns and monks live very well. Their lives are still full of love and, as they would say, when freed from the obligation to love mainly one person, their love extends equally to all. The response is that they are deeply loved by many souls in return.

But find me someone who has regular sex without love and is truly happy. Could we find such a person? So it felt very beautiful and very appropriate to end our weekend with a process that wasn't about sex at all but about emotional connection. It would be sad, I guess, to have a couples' workshop and not send the couples home as friends. If you'd like to take your partner to this workshop, the link is in the Notes at the end.[9]

We finished our thank yous and goodbyes and piled our stuff in a cab to get the train back to London. T had done something that no man has ever done for me before. Not much more expensive but a sweet surprise: after a weekend about sex, an appreciative boyfriend had booked us first class seats home.

'And I'm happy to do it again,' he said.

'Really?'

'Whenever we spend the weekend away exploring sex, I'll pay and we can travel home first class. I appreciate a woman who thinks a good sex life is important.'

I think many men would say this if they experienced this work.

Long Hot Summer

Stroking the Clitoris

I have been reading a book called *The Multi-Orgasmic Couple* by Mantak Chia. As you may imagine, it's seriously annoying. How many multi-orgasmic couples do you think you know? What is most annoying is that, for the man, there are exercises about how to separate the orgasm from the ejaculation so that he can then orgasm as often as he'd like to. That process, although difficult for the man to achieve, is a physical one. The advice for women starts with asking the woman to go back to her childhood and examine how she feels about every formative sexual experience. I have become somewhat weary of this approach. It seems to be such a frequent assumption that if a woman isn't orgasmic she is messed up and needs to work through her 'issues' in an exhaustive and detailed way. And often, historically, with a male therapist.

The Multi-Orgasmic Couple is yet another book with a male analysis of female sexuality. As we know, a woman, when examined by a man, is often just too complex. If she's not responsive in the same way he is, men often declare us broken. It's all Freud's fault. And Jung didn't really help either.

I call Hilly and complain. 'Don't read that book,' she says with admirable clarity, 'it does have a very male perspective.

Read *Slow Sex* by Nicole Daedone.'

I go to my local bookshop and order this (great title) and, when it arrives, I'm not in the least annoyed. There is no suggestion here that if you want a good sex life you need to turn your psyche inside out or consider the first time you saw a penis. It's cleverly and empathetically written. Nicole's writing on 'what a woman wants from a man' and 'what a man wants from a woman' is so compassionate that both T and I fall a little in love with Nicole when we read it. But the most amazing thing about the book is one simple exercise that it describes ... now, pay attention.

The key process in Nicole's book is what she calls 'Orgasmic Meditation'. They call it OMing. As OM is the most sacred sound in Hinduism and is also found in Jainism, Sikhism and Buddhism, I'm not sure whether to cringe when they call it 'The OM practice' or admire their marketing. Anyway, this is what they do. The man carefully makes a 'nest' on the floor with blankets and cushions. The woman removes her clothing from the waist down and lies on the floor with her legs butterflied to reveal her 'pussy' (change of vocabulary here – she doesn't use the word 'yoni'). The cushions support her left leg. He sits down beside her on her right. He is fully clothed. His body supports her right leg. His left leg is over her tummy. The position is complicated to describe but is easy to get into.[10] Then, get this! He is to spend the next 15 minutes stroking the upper left-hand quadrant of her clitoris with a stroke no firmer than that which you would use to stroke your own eyelid. That's it. I remember feeling slightly faint when I first read this.

Nicole has thought of everything. His ideal hand position is described. The man (or woman in a same-sex relationship) gently opens the labial lips to reveal the clitoris fully. Then he uses the thumb and second finger of his left hand to hold the lips open (and the hood back.) Then, with the first finger of the left hand the stroker simply learns to stroke the clitoris. He places the thumb of his right hand at the base of her introitus (entrance to her vaginal canal) and rests it there lightly but assuredly. It's a very subtle process and it seems that Nicole has considered and found a solution for every possible difficulty that could come up. For example, for women who have trouble giving direction and who would experience difficulty saying, 'I think you need to move a fraction to the right,' she has the man ask questions to which the woman simply replies 'yes' or 'no'. So a stroker might ask, 'Would you like me to move a little to the right?' Or, 'Would you like a firmer stroke?' Or even simply, 'A different stroke?'

For the stroker who may be doing their best, and a braver strokee, she has a way for the person being stroked to give feedback that is not discouraging. So first you find something that is good, and then add a request to it. So it may sound like this: 'Pressure feels good – a little faster please.' Or, 'Position feels good – a little lighter please.' So Nicole has worked out a simple set of guidelines to make the communication between the partners as easy as possible.

It's like learning to play a musical instrument. The stroker learns slowly but surely by feeling empathetically the result of the strokes on the woman. The truly liberating aspect of this practice is that it is not goal-oriented. In other words, the stroker is not trying to produce an orgasm in the woman. The only instructions to the person being stroked are 'relax and open'. That's it.

This idea fascinates me for several reasons: Firstly, it's an easy, incredibly easy, way to focus on learning how to give pleasure to the woman. As we all know it is usually far easier for a man to receive pleasure from a woman than the other way around, so this seems like a practice that is well overdue. Secondly, it's so simple; it doesn't begin by asking me whether my earliest experiences were traumatic or assume that I am repressed or dysfunctional in some way. It's simply lie down, open your legs, relax and enjoy. Thirdly, it's about concentrating on sensation; whatever the sensation is, without judging it or pushing for more.

I'm almost perspiring with a mixture of terror and anticipation – just reading it. What the book describes is a long journey that both the stroker and the strokee go through. The stroker learns how to tune into the body of the woman. A man isn't necessarily intuitive to the high levels of sensitivity that the clitoris seems to demand and a woman isn't necessarily able to receive the pleasure that her clitoris can give her. So you learn together. And there are all kinds of promises, of a feeling of 'electricity' that the man can have travelling through his finger and through his body that comes from the woman. A woman being able to experience sensations more extraordinary and powerful than any ordinary orgasm can give. The book also speaks of this practice as being a source of energy for the woman and a powerfully empowering experience for the man. And some couples spend their evenings watching television?

I want to pluck up the courage to ask T to read the book and consider becoming my 'stroker'. I order a second copy and sit down to write a letter. Later he suggests I copy the letter to you in full.

Dearest T

I can honestly say that out of all the scary things I've done in my life, giving you this book is the scariest. It feels like entrusting you with my whole life. That is not overstating it – you'll see why as you read.

I place myself in your hands, grateful that your hands are capable, your spirit is willing and your heart is pure. Please know that it is not the strong confident woman who knows how to take care of you when you're having a bad day, but a far younger and more vulnerable part of me speaking. But don't worry, she comes to you willingly and all she wants is fifteen minutes of your time. Often.

Please be sensitive around this book and don't crack jokes about it. 'Normal' sex is easier to combine with humour and maybe we will laugh if you are willing to travel this journey with me – but at first, just as the book says, it's about safety and this requires more vulnerability than I'm accustomed to.

For my part, if you are willing to read and to do this with me – I promise to take the best care of your heart and your body that I am able.

So please read and let me know. Are you willing to learn all this with me and to be with me through the 'ups' and the 'downs'?

I am breathing and waiting for your answer.

With fear and joy, xx Isabel

T said,

'That was a really beautiful letter. I've read it about 25 times ... So it's a sort of mixture of sex and meditation? Single point of focus, but instead of focusing on the breath I'm asked to focus on your clitoris?'

'Yes, you could say that. Or on the sensation on the tip of your finger when it's touching my clitoris.'

'And I have to keep my clothes on?'

'Yes.'

'And look between your legs and not become aroused?'

'As I understand it there is nothing wrong with you being aroused but the point is to channel the arousal correctly. Before you start the practice you are asked to describe what you see but using descriptive, not evaluative, language.'

'Why's that?'

'Because if you say to many women, "You're beautiful," they may not believe you. Many women have ambivalent feelings about their yoni, er – pussy. But if you say, "You have a darker shade of flesh on the inner lips than on the outer lips and your inner lips fan out slightly more to the left than to the right and make a petal shape," or something like that, then no woman can argue with you because you are just describing what you are seeing and not putting a value on it. I can see that this would work to help women accept what the man is describing.'

'So I'm not allowed to tell you that, as a man, I find what I see beautiful?'

'Nope.'

'And that makes sense to you?'

'Absolutely. T, would you read the book?'

'My other reading has been put aside. It's been thrown out of the window.'

So T reads and agrees, enthusiastically, to become a student of the Orgasmic Meditation practice.

'I've read the first four chapters. Can we start now?'

'No. Please read the rest of the book.'

He was keen.

He created an evening when we had 15 minutes. The time demand being so small is really helpful. As the woman you don't feel that you're being overly demanding. The practice encourages the couple to have the 'nest' away from the bedroom and to keep this practice entirely free from the rest of your sex life. Nervously we set up cushions on the floor, some rugs covered with a towel to lie on. We had acquired some basic lube as we decided that the £15 official lube that came with the programme online was overpriced and probably just coconut oil anyway. Then we attempted to find the correct position, both feeling rather clumsy and awkward.

'Does my leg go here?'

'Ow! No, that can't be right.'

We fumbled around.

'It says that we need a light so that I can see clearly.'

'OK, so put the extra light on.'

'And if I put my iPhone on 15 minutes that should work.'

'OK.'

'What sound do you want at the end? A car horn? Space travel?'

'I don't think so. The harp please.'

'Hold on.' He got up again.

'OK. Well, I'll lie down then.'

'Is it too cold in here?'

'Yes. Can we put the heater on?'

'Are you OK with that cushion?'

'No. I don't want one with a donkey looking at me on it. It seems weird somehow. Please give me a cushion without a face.'

'OK. Can I lean my back against the sofa do you think?'

'Yes, it's important that you are comfortable all the time.'

'Is this cushion the right height for me to sit on?'

'No, pass the Zafu.'

And so ... eventually ... we started our first Orgasmic Meditation.

Afterwards we took out pen and paper. I wrote,

Session One

God, I was scared. Why would it be so scary to open my legs and have a man stroke my clitoris? But he was so gentle that he stopped it being scary. T admits that he really doesn't know where anything is – which is understandable because, based on precision of feeling alone, neither do I.

At first when he started – beautifully softly – it felt as though he was stroking the outside of the hood rather than the most sensitive area. It felt good though and I wasn't sure whether to re-direct him or not. He was tender with his touch and it felt warm. I did feel gentle warmth through my body. I wondered if he needed to hold the hood back further or whether my clit wasn't erect. (Honestly, I really feel as if I ought to have more understanding of my own body.) And it felt as if we needed a little more lube ... Fantastically moved that he is willing to do this with me. Position felt comfortable. Clit still feels slightly warm. Appreciative of the attention.

T wrote,

Easy. Comfortable. I'm a bit clueless about the clit. How to find it precisely and how to stroke in the manner that we are supposed to. Isabel was great – not nervous the way she thought she would be. Or at least, didn't let on. She was willing to try. To be. To allow.

I didn't feel clumsy – rather just clueless. Hard to open her with just thumb and second finger and stroke with the index finger. The index finger needs to be soft and mobile and the other fingers firm.

This was definitely one of the most extraordinary things I've done in my life so far. But a practice that requires only 15 minutes isn't hard to find time for. After Session Two I wrote,

T was concentrating on the outer lips and I really wanted him to pull back the hood and say 'Oh, that's where it is and what it looks like' – so that he could enlighten me too. I mean, I've seen it but it's not as if I look in a mirror regularly to examine the details. T experimented with stroking on slightly different positions today. It's hard to guide him because when he first touched the tip of the clit I said, 'Please don't touch there, it's too sensitive.' And then later I wanted him to. There were times when he was stroking when there was a wonderful heat in me that made my hands and nipples tingle and at other times I felt absolutely numb. It's very hard for me not to enter into self-judgement at these times and feel that I 'should' be responding differently. I even found myself worrying about T's finger. As if he can't look after himself. But then there are moments when I do remember to breathe and just go back to focusing on the sensation. It's wonderful when a beautifully subtle sensation fills my body that comes directly from the stroking and it sometimes takes a couple of hours to subside.

It's scary but I wish I knew whether T is stroking the hood or the clit itself. Look forward to being able to be sure of the difference.

And he didn't write anything ... the children returned from school. Sometimes real life takes over. Fifteen minutes is really 30 minutes by the time you've laid out the 'nest', calmed down, had an optional hug, done the practice and tidied away. But it's still easy to fit into the day.

We made time daily; neither of us in much of a hurry but just happy to have found this practice – a different way of enjoying time. A bit like sex, yet not like sex. A bit like meditation, yet not much like meditation.

We bought the official 'OneTaste' lube and found, after all, that it was worth the money. Coconut Oil is very good for massage and, er, other practices, and many of the commercial lubes are horrible. For this practice you need something with the right viscosity. They hand-make theirs out of olive oil, beeswax, shea butter and grapeseed oil and use only organic ingredients. As they use it every day they obviously care a lot about the feel of it. So, if you want to have a go at all this I recommend getting their lube.[11]

After session 12 I wrote,

Today there was a moment when T and I really felt for the first time the tip of his finger on my clitoris. I'm seriously beginning to worry that I may have an exceptionally small clitoris as T seems to be having such trouble finding precisely the right point but Nicole's book says that it's common for the man to have trouble. We women have so many folds of flesh and the clitoris can be elusive – it appears and then disappears again. And, like a subtle creature that retreats into itself, it seems, it/she needs to be lured out and can retreat and vanish again with surprising speed if the pressure is wrong.

It has been very hard for me to give direction and to communicate. Even when it's going well it's hard for me to guide him. Today T broke with the guidelines in the book and gave a direct instruction. 'Just breathe and relax,' he said. So I did. A bit. I know my job is to 'open to sensation' as Nicole calls it. 'Just focus on sensation.' But even that feels hard.

There was a moment today when it did feel like very delicate waves of light going through me. A very gentle sensation and a beautiful one.

What is so delicious about the feeling of T's finger in contact is how subtle it is. And he felt it too today ... just a little. I am so grateful to him for being prepared to go on this journey with me.

Meanwhile T was writing too. He wrote after that session,

Feeling more confident. Perhaps. Able to find my way around the many layers of skin. I need to breathe. I need to get more feedback. Seeing how this could be important for us. For her – sure. But maybe for us too. Maybe this practice addresses some of my issues of connection and vulnerability. Need to lean forward and really see. Need to go in deeper but equally be soft.

And my notes after our 14th practice read,

One of the things that these sessions are bringing up for me is how scared I am. Despite the fact that it's always pleasurable – there is a part of me that dreads them as if I were anticipating a dental appointment. Once they start they are always lovely so I have to wonder why I almost do my best to avoid them. I realize that I'm unaccustomed to feeling that what is between my legs is a source of pleasure – it has been more a source of grief. My primary associations with the word 'vagina' would be 'blood', 'pain', 'cystitis', 'birth' and these words would all come before 'pleasure'. And I suppose a source of pleasure for men, less for me. So this, which is for the woman's pleasure is an alien experience. How absurd that this should be so.

I believe that I offered a line of feedback in the correct format. 'That pressure feels about right. Could you try a little further to the right?' It's SO subtle though. I'm encouraged by Nicole's instruction in her book: 'see if you can feel just one stroke'. Because I focus on that and I can feel always feel one.

Just as with a musical instrument, you may not be able to play skilfully but from the very first lesson, if you are well taught and you concentrate, you can make a beautiful sound from the first note; so it is with this practice.

• • •

T and I are not living together, so we can't practise every day as they recommend, but we are managing two or three orgasmic meditation sessions a week. We kept referring to the book and I kept doing my research and then I found out that the author, Nicole, was coming to London to give a talk. I already loved her from her writing. I found her loving, brave, tender and empowering.

I wrote to her and asked for an interview. I offered to

change all my plans in order to see her and, much to my delight, she agreed. I played with the 'record' button on my iPhone and set off, joyfully, to meet the woman who had written this amazing book and brought this whole new experience into my life. On my own and on behalf of all of us, I had a few questions for her.

An Interview with the Clit Whisperer – Nicole Daedone

I arrive in a smart, white, flat that some clever person had rented for Nicole on her visit to London. Nicole is the founder of 'OneTaste' – which teaches OMing internationally – and her staff know how to take care of her.

Nicole doesn't walk. She moves with a mixture of a glide and a bound. She is an astoundingly beautiful, healthy and sexy woman, and she celebrates and enjoys that. But it's not about her having a big ego. I didn't feel from her any of the 'I'm impressive, aren't I?' feeling that you get with people who look great but underneath are insecure and so are trying to impress you. Nicole felt free from needing to think about herself. She's done her work on herself and today was meeting me so she put all her concentration on my needs in the interview. It's easy to tell that she has done her spiritual work as well as her sexual work. She had nothing to prove; she isn't concerned about how my impressions may reflect on her, she's just having fun. She's like an Afghan Hound – friendly, but not attached; enjoying you but not collecting you;

interested but not judgemental; informative but not preachy. I'd enjoyed her book so much I was afraid that she might not live up to my expectations but instead she exceeded them. It is rare to meet someone so free. I didn't have to explain anything. I could just get on with the interview. So I did. I sat on her white sofa and ate too many of her raspberries.

'Nicole, I'd like to get straight to the key questions, if I may? Life is short after all.'

'Yes it is.'

'So – about orgasms ...'

She laughed.

I wasn't beating about the bush. 'There are a lot of people that I've met in the course of my journey that are still telling me that real orgasms are vaginal. Your emphasis is the clitoris; can you tell me why please? Didn't Freud teach that little girls like the clitoris and big girls like the vagina?'

Nicole smiles her huge smile and starts chatting, as if to her best friend, with her Californian accent. 'I think all orgasm is clitoral. Whether it's the back of the clitoris or the front. What's important is the point of access and the point that you want is the bit where we know that 8,000 nerve endings are bundled. There's a spot that we are directing our partner to if we say "a little bit to the left or the right". That spot, for me, is where you plug into the body of a woman.'

'All women?'

Naomi Wolf wrote in her book *Vagina* that women have different neural pathways and this leads to some having more nerve endings around the clitoris, and, according to Naomi anyway, some in different areas of the vagina, the perineum or the anus.

I get that, 'All women?' question a lot. Some women even say, 'I'm pretty sure it's not me.' And so we have them do our practice starting wherever they think they feel most and then trying this spot and time after time it comes back to this spot in the upper left hand quadrant. I have never worked with a woman who has not had that spot light up.

'How long have you been doing this work with women?'

'Over 15 years.'

'And how many women do you think you've seen in that time?'

'Thousands.'

It's hard not to be impressed.

'How I feel about everything is: try it and see for yourself. Keep an open mind to a different possibility. I had good sex when I started all this but it was as if I'd been really good at aerobics and then I started yoga and there was this whole other dimension that was available. Previously I'd not even know that it existed. So I was shocked open.'

It's hard not to like the sound of this. I can't say that I had yet been 'shocked open'. But I'd had glimmers of possibilities.

'Very good, Nicole. So, "try it and see". And how would you describe "it" exactly?'

'You stroke the clitoris. That's about it. The woman lies down. The partner strokes the upper left hand quadrant of the clitoris. "Up, down – up, down – up, down." No more firmly than you would stroke an eyelid. For 15 minutes.'

'No one can complain that it's complicated, can they?'

'They can't. And it's goal-less. We take the whole goal of reaching, striving for the climax away. The only thing to do is to feel. And as simple as it is, for many women – it ends up being the most profound experience that they've ever had.'

I'm glad she said '... ends up being'. 'But it takes practice, doesn't it? Just the same way breathing meditation does.'

'It's exactly the same with breathing meditation. You do this simple thing of focusing on your breath. Yet people do it for years to levels of unbelievable mastery. This is like that.'

'Wonderful.'

Hard not to love the idea of being played like an instrument with a skill of 'unbelievable mastery'. But what about the vagina?

'I've been reading Naomi Wolf's book, *Vagina*, as I said, and she has interviewed a number of psycho-sexual experts. She puts forward the view that there is a direct connection between the vagina and the brain. I understand that the body is all connected and everywhere is wired to the brain but she is saying, specifically if I have understood her correctly, that your earliest sexual experiences are formative in the way that your body gets mapped.'

'Mmmm?' Nicole is a much better listener than I am. I always interrupt whereas Nicole actually listens.

'I was quite depressed by that because I started my sex life with a bad marriage and I think I numbed out a lot. So when I read her book I thought "Oh shit" because if that's "mapped" and can't be un-mapped then I'm a lost cause.'

'Does she say that there is no way that the damage can be undone?'

'She doesn't state it directly but she certainly seems to suggest that a lot of the mapping is extremely formative. For example, in people who have been victims of sexual abuse or have been raped, she appeared to be suggesting that once the neural pathways are set up, we have been "programmed" a certain way....'

'Ooo, I have some thoughts on this,' Nicole replied enthusiastically. 'Have you heard of neuro-plasticity?'

'I read a book called *The Brain That Changes Itself*. It's an inspiring book about the brain's ability to re-wire itself after trauma.'

'I'm a strong believer because I've witnessed it time and time again with this repeated practice. I think one of the primary reasons that you don't see a lot of growth in a woman's sexuality, if she has trauma, is that you don't see any practices that actually reverse trauma. Look at the way many people view sex ... under the covers, in the dark without talking. And then, as a woman, no matter what, I'm supposed to enjoy it. And if I don't I'm still supposed to act like I do. Well, surely that can cause trauma? That's terrible.'

I hope you have a taste for the black humour of the reality of many women's lives here?

'That makes sense. Terrible sense.'

'Do you know the work of Dr Lori Brotto?'

'Not yet.'

'She looks at how mindfulness practices in terms of orgasm actually begin to shift the body. My experience has been that when you slowly and incrementally introduce change and you work with a woman's body in a way where her body gets to direct how it goes – that experience begins to undo what may have been done. That's the first part.'

'Hmm.' I say articulately.

'The second part: the way I look at it – every woman's mapping is beautiful and I seek to honour that with the practice and work with it. We often find that a lot of trauma ends up being fuel for awakening in terms of a woman's orgasm.'

'So you disagree that the programming is set?'

'We say – "start where you are". We notice that, progressively and incrementally, it gets better.'

This was good news. If people who have never had pleasure can learn to have pleasure, then there is hope for every woman who has a clitoris and wants to learn how to receive pleasure from it. And you don't have to go to a therapist and talk about penis envy or things that happened to you as a child – you can grow through practising pleasure. What do you think of that, Sigmund?

'I heard a story that you worked with a couple that hadn't touched for 17 years.'

'Eighteen actually. You want to know the terrifying thing? That's common. I'd say that 50% of the couples that I work with enter and are sitting on opposite sides of the sofa. They don't even know how to have that simple uncomplicated intimacy with each other. They've lost that. I think it's because we've all been told that sex in marriage is supposed to be "natural".'

'Yes.'

'Natural and spontaneous and everyone's supposed to

know how to do it and how to maintain it. It progressively dies out and we all seem to agree that if you've been together a long time that part of your relationship is going to die.'

'That seems to be the most usual thinking.'

'I refuse to believe that.'

It's hard not to love this woman.

'Good for you. So do I.'

'I just taught at a university. There were 500 students in the auditorium and at one point in the evening a young girl stood up. She was trembling, and in a very shaky voice said, "Er, Ms Daedone – will you just make sure that all the men know where the clitoris is?" She was right. So I showed them a picture and said, "This is where the clitoris is." And I watched the guys looking shocked. So, just being exactly sure where to find it is pretty important information.'

I told her my favourite joke, and the story that I opened the book with, about the 53-year-old taxi driver. We sighed.

'So, what about you?' Nicole asked.

'Me?'

'Yes, you.' Nicole smiled at me. I was obviously not going to get out easily.

'Well, my partner and I have been doing the practice and I've noticed a shift in me from, "Oh my goodness, do I really want to do this? I'm sure I have some emails that I have to attend to ..." to, at the end of the practice, saying to my partner, "This feels really good. Can you remind me that I really enjoy this?" So I look forward to it. But I'm running judgement on myself that I'm not having enough sensation.'

'Say more?'

Aghhhh. Run away!

'I find giving feedback to my partner hard as I'm sometimes not sure what direction I want to give.'

'It's a common problem for women.'

'I like the exercise where the man asks questions and all the woman has to say is, "yes" or "no". I love that. So if he says, "Would you like me to move to a firmer stroke?" I can manage to say "yes" or "no" although it's still hard not to add "please and thank you" and "if it's not too much trouble" in a British kind of way.'

'Does it seem too much trouble to your partner?'

'Not at all. He loves the practice. But I tell myself that somehow my sensation should be greater than it is.'

Basically, I should be hanging from the ceiling screaming with pleasure instead of lying contentedly on the floor enjoying the subtlest of sensation.

'Yes, many women start with the idea that they are somehow doing it wrong. I tell the story about my first session ... the fact is that all we are supposed to do is lie there ... All I have to do is lie down ... that's it. It's a goal-less practice. And I'm thinking, "I'm not turning him on. I'm not doing this right." I remember actually thinking, "I'm not feeling enough. This should be deeper. I should be trembling ..." I had all these ideas about what I thought my experience should be. I couldn't find my damned orgasm.'

'When you say "orgasm", you don't mean climax – you mean the entire orgasmic response?'

Nicole distinguishes between a climax – which is not

where the practice puts the priority, and all other sensation. In this practice they call the entire experience of arousal your orgasm.

'Right. What happens with the practice is that you get to experience. I have women that come to me and they say, "I didn't feel anything." I work with them on what I call the "green leaf" process.'

'Yes, you write about just feeling one stroke. The green leaf process is focusing on the sensation one stroke at a time?'

'Yes. And if you can do that then you can go the whole 15 minutes focusing on sensation.'

'Yup.'

'Women come to me and say, "I didn't feel anything".' I say, 'Nothing at all?' And they say, 'Well, there was this one moment where I saw God.'

'I haven't seen God but I enjoy the subtlety of just feeling one stroke properly and I enjoy the sensitivity of your writing and your understanding of what is a private and inner process. So I love it ... so far.'

Yes, I can honestly say that it's the most wonderful and most weird sexual practice ever.

'On behalf of my readers who may be thinking, "What about the man?" I have lots of girlfriends who I think would love to do this practice but they may be thinking, "I certainly couldn't do this with my current partner," or, "I can't find a partner." And my question would be, "Does the partner matter?" The reason I ask this is that I know a tantra teacher called Hilly who is the person who recommended your book to me. She has had six different fathers of her six children. And I asked her, "When you were with father number six, did you sometimes find yourself missing father number two?" She said to me, "After a while I realized that they are all just different faces of the same God".'

Nicole gasped with delight. 'That's a high-level practice. In yoga they teach beginning, intermediate and advanced. And I think that in the beginning it matters that he is safe and trusted. Because if he isn't then your vigilance centre can't go down.'

'The "vigilance centre" is the part of your brain that is always on the lookout for you, checking that you are safe?'

'Right. So you need to have someone that you feel safe with so that you can relax fully. A lot of women come to me and say, "What should I do?" and I tell them that when I first started the practice I didn't have a boyfriend and so I called my ex and I said, "Look, we're not going to get back together but would you like to try this practice?" Because I knew that I trusted him and I knew that he was safe. And we still have a practice – 14 years later. And we still aren't romantic. But it's a very deep and very intimate relationship. It's a high-level practice to have the perspective that Hilly has – to see all men as different faces of the same God. I believe that ultimately her perspective is the truth. But in the beginning I say to women, start with someone who is safe. It certainly doesn't have to be anyone who you feel is "the one".'

I'm so bored of hearing this myth that there is one man or woman out there for us. I was surprised to hear the words 'the one' come out of Nicole's mouth. As Tim Minchin says in his great song 'If I Didn't Have You',[12] it's just statistically unlikely that out of 999,999 possible lovers there is just one who is designed for us. And then of course you have to believe in a conscious universe ... a power that would then be responsible, logically, for all the bad things that happen to us.

'Isn't "the one" a Hollywood romantic myth, Nicole? Don't you think?'

'My feeling is "yes and no". And I don't know that there is a "the one" but I do know that, rather like when I had my first orgasmic meditation and I had an experience where something exponentially shifted – where I saw an entirely different location ... Well, I know that that is possible with someone. You know the saying "phase transition" – where water is ice and then it melts and it turns to water, and then it evaporates? Well, you can have a phase transition experience with someone. It's not just the next person who you fall in love with but someone who gives you a profoundly different experience of life.'

'Ah, yes.' I sighed. 'Meanwhile I can imagine my reader friends reading this and thinking, "I can't see Bert doing this." But, as you write so beautifully Nicole, all men want to please their women and often they don't have a clue. Like the taxi driver I spoke of.'

'One of the reasons that we have de-coupled it from a lot of different societal notions is that you achieve a level of human connection without all the stories. And so you might be with "Bert", your husband of 15 years, and maybe you're not feeling super romantic with him ... But that place of human connection – you can find it with OM and it nourishes you no matter what.'

'Yes.'

'But surely, to want to go this deeply you would only want to do this with ... er ... someone that you wanted to go this deeply with.' I said, articulately.

'Not necessarily. It's a big deal to want to lie down and have "lovemaking". I mean, you kind of have to have some kind of romantic feelings to do that, but to OM you can be doing the dishes one minute and then lie down and have plain nourishing human connection and then get up and finish the dishes. That for me is one of the beauties of the practice. You don't have to feel that you're in love, you don't have to put any lingerie on, you don't have to have this big story ... you can just "be" with your partner.'

'You don't have to be in love with Bert then? Or anyone you stroke with or are stroked by?'

'You don't.'

'Why would any woman want to have such a profound experience with a man that they are not in love with?'

'I think there are a number of reasons ...'

'Actually, I know the answer.'

I could hardly have been doing spiritual work for years and not know the answer.

Nicole smiles at me again excitedly. 'What? I want to know what you think.'

'As the spiritual teachers always tell us ... the real journey is with yourself.'

'You got it.'

So women, not one of us is broken. We just need to be
handled right. And how to get to be handled right? Well,
that is up to us. And men? Well, I certainly hope that there
is no other skill that you'd rather have. I mean, surely this
is better than making money or playing football? This is
the power to make women very happy. This is a skill you
learn and then apply to all your lovemaking. The skill
of awareness, connection and focus. This is becoming a
sexual magician.

• • •

As I left, Nicole suggested that we might be interested in
having private lessons. Can you imagine? T and I could go
to the home of a woman in London and she would coach
us both. Is your mind boggling? I've been teaching for
years the value of doing what scares you. So I must walk
my talk. We have been doing the practice for months now
and, to keep the analogy of the musical instrument going,
I don't want to get into any bad habits and maybe this
woman would have just the tip we need to deepen the
practice. T was less scared than I was about this. He made
the appointment.

'And I paid too.' He tells me later when I read this back
to him.

And he bought the future teacher a convertible. Well,
he didn't, but I'm sure he would have done if he'd had the
money spare. Just to make really sure he was going to get
her best attention.

Taking Lessons: How to Stroke and Be Stroked

A normal-looking house with a normal-looking door, but ringing the bell is a bit like seeing a therapist. After all we are here to have some aspect of our behaviour adjusted. The lady we are seeing is Justine Dawson. She is a slim, attractive blonde in her 40s who trained with Nicole in the US and is now in London teaching. She shows us into a small room and we sit and start to chat. Or at least, I talk a lot.

'... And I'm beginning to think that perhaps I have the smallest clitoris in the Western world,' I confide. 'Even when looking closely, T sometimes can't find it and I have no idea how to direct him. The most sensitive upper left quadrant of the clitoris that you speak of seems to move?'

'Don't you mean upper right?' says T.

'I guess it's upper right for you but it's upper left for me when I'm lying down so I think of it as the upper left position – 1pm on the clock face.'

I talk, eager to avoid the more practical part of the lesson. This is like going to a music lesson and wasting time telling the teacher about your instrument.

'If you'd like to lie down, Isabel? I'll just check the position you are both in.'

She's so matter of fact. Just relax, Isabel. Have to ignore the 'WTF are you doing?' questions racing around my mind. Just stop thinking. Breathe. I can't believe I'm doing this.

'You need to make sure that there is no strain on your back,' she says to T.

'Isabel, would you like another cushion?'

'Yes, please.'

'It's important that the woman has enough support. You need to be 100% comfortable.'

'OK.' I try to keep breathing. I try to relax. Contradiction. Yes, I know.

They look at the matter in hand. 'And there is Isabel's perfectly normal-sized clitoris.' Justine says.

I laugh. What a relief. Bless Justine for that observation. I wonder if I'm really going to write about this later.

'If you take the lube?' She and T discuss finger positions and the angle of the arm – just as if he were playing a cello.

'Be sure to give at least one instruction. OK, Isabel?'

'OK.' She's so practical about it all. Amazing.

T says, 'I'm going to touch you now,' as the practice requires. This is so that the strokee can relax fully and nothing surprising happens, which would startle you and raise the vigilance centre in the brain and so prevent relaxation.

They discuss more or less lube and then he begins to stroke.

'A little bit further up and to the right – just a tiny fraction,' Justine says.

I feel more in tune.

'And if you just adjust the angle of your finger so you are slightly more on the tip.'

I feel more sensation.

'And if you could give an instruction, Isabel?'

'Er – that feels like a good position. If you could just stay there.' I manage to enunciate.

I have no idea where the 15 minutes goes. I lie there feeling very light and happy while they discuss technique in a goal-less practice. This was certainly the weirdest experience of my life. So far. But it was wonderful. When the time was up we thanked Justine as if we had just been for any other kind of consultation. And walked out into the street as if it was all a dream. I was in a kind of exhilarated shock.

'Good grief. I need a coffee. What did we just do?'

'That was amazing, weird and, in a bizarre way, really wonderful,' said T.

The following morning our usual practice was noticeably improved. Not that we have a goal of course. It just felt more, well – in tune.

• • •

We had just got used to the idea of being coached when Justine phones and asked if we'd like to join the London 'OM Circle'. If you are in a relationship there is nothing to stop you using this practice exclusively with your partner. But they had yet more on offer. An entire community, previously unknown to me, has grown up around Nicole and the book. People who wanted to learn the OM practice found each other. People who had been practising a long time started to teach people who were new. Those who wanted to practise every day even moved in together and created OM community houses. And then some of this came to London. So in Central London (and by the time you read this they may be in a town near you) there is something called an 'OM Circle'. No, really, I am not making this up. Groups of people who would like either to learn to be very good at stroking a clitoris or very good at knowing how to relax so that they can enjoy having their clitoris stroked – meet. You just have to go for a training session or attend a training day and then you can go to a group OM practice. The links are at the end of the book so you can consider whether you'd like to try any of this.

It sounds bizarre doesn't it? But what it offers, for men, is the opportunity to learn how another clitoris responds to the stroke and for the strokee – well, me, the chance to be stroked by a different stroker with a different energy, and hopefully to learn something from that experience about receiving. Each evening has two 15-minute practices. If you go to the practice with a regular partner you have the option of either staying together for both sessions or having one session with your partner and one session with someone else.

'But can't you learn with just your partner?'

'Yes, you can. But if you have a similar experience at each OM session, how do you know whether it's you who is stuck or your partner?'

I toyed with the idea of holding interviews and auditions. 'To apply, please send details of how many years' practice you have. And please send a photograph along with a short essay, in less than 1,000 words, on why the OM practice is of interest to you and what you feel you could bring to this opportunity.' But it doesn't work like that. Sadly.

Is this all beginning to sound a little dodgy to you? Well, it's certainly outside the box, isn't it? And I can hear questions in the ether – let me answer just one of them. 'What about hygiene?' And the answer is that they have super-thin gloves that they use, once only of course, and everyone uses them unless they are touching their regular partner.

At first, I had no interest in going. The invitation horrified me. Neither Justine, nor another leading London teacher called Rachel who organizes these events, called more than once. The OM Circles are free so no one is making money from these nights. The option is just there to teach, learn and enrich your practice. But as the weeks went by – inevitably I suppose, I began to be curious. I teach the value of going outside the comfort zone. It's a way of life that I believe in – continually challenging ourselves. I love what T and I are doing. I love the way that he strokes. But I'm still having difficulty knowing how to give him instructions. My perception of where he strokes me and where I'd like him to stroke more, or less – is vague. And I'm keen to learn. Maybe – if I become, briefly, the instrument of a man who is a more experienced stroker then I, as the instrument, may learn something valuable that I could then feedback to T?

I tell him about the circle and T goes white – I see this clearly even though he's at the other end of the phone. But, as always on this journey, nervous but excited, he agrees. And he's fine, until we arrive. Outside in the car, he goes into high anxiety.

'I am experiencing more anticipation, excitement and utter dread before our chosen activity tonight than anything I've done in recent memory,' T communicates with clarity. 'I mean – I've thought about this and it's another man touching my girlfriend. It's taken us a long time to get here. You've allowed me, with a lot of initial trepidation, to go to a tender and gentle divinity in you. What's happened to the sacredness of tantra?'

'I don't know. I don't see this as less sacred. Perhaps I've done too much spiritual work. I see everything as sacred.' But T wasn't listening ... he was talking.

'On the other hand I ask myself, "I'm a bloke and I get to stroke another woman. So what's my problem?"'

I breathe in but before I can answer he goes on.
'I'll tell you what my problem is. These are men and men want sex. You are beautiful and I'm sure you could go home with any of the men who are there.'

'I don't think so, T. The majority will be there with their partners and I think it's reasonable to assume that they like their own women better than a stranger. I'm going home with you. And why do you assume that the second OM stroker will necessarily be better than you?'

My answers weren't relevant. His objections went on.

'But this is your most tender essence.'

'Darling boyfriend – we don't have to do this if you don't want to.'

'No, we're here now so we may as well go in. Just remind me, why are we doing this?'

'To learn. To learn about ourselves, each other and sexual energy.'

'I have another fear,' he said without pausing for breath. 'I'm afraid that maybe it will be good for you. Or for me even. Why would we rock the boat? Why would we want to know what's out there? My sexual relations with you are the best that I've ever had. Why would I want to endanger that?'

'You can walk away if you want to. We can walk away if you'd like us to. I'm not attached to this. I'm just intrigued.'

'Yes, but I'm also intrigued. I booked the session after all. I've driven us here. I've even found a parking place, dammit. We're here. Why do we need other people to help us become better lovers? Can't we do this on our own?'

'Maybe we can. Maybe we can't. Maybe it's just faster like this.'

'I'm afraid that some other man will stroke you better or that you'll want to come back and I won't. After all, there is more in this for you. You are getting stroked. I love your clitoris. I've looked at it a lot in the last couple of months. And when we go home I will not be the last guy to have touched you. And he doesn't belong there. Unless you want him there. I mean, it's your body.'

Do I want him there? I don't even know who 'he' is. There is clarity in that he's just an anonymous male. 'Do you want to do this or not?'

'No. Yes. No. Yes. Oh, come on. I've paid for the parking.'

So in we went.

• • •

In a rather beautiful studio, which is perhaps more traditionally used for ballet classes, was a room covered with yoga mats, cushions and a large number of very attractive people.

'Goodness, T. Everyone here is beautiful.' I guess to be here you have, at the least, the courage to go after what you want and either a relationship or the determination to find one. To be a man here you have to have a genuine desire to want to learn to please women. And to be a woman alone here – well, that's courage. They all seem to have an almost vibrant positive energy. I don't know why. It's not as if I had consciously expected this gathering to be filled with the kind of low-energy people that I more often meet at spiritual gatherings (very loving but maybe slightly depressed) but this is quite different. For one thing there is an equal number of men and women. The organizers make sure of that. I have no idea how. I suppose no single man wants to cross London and then find that all the women are taken and no single woman wants to cross London in anticipation of a new experience and not have one.

A woman says, 'Raise your hand if you need a number two for tonight.' T and I both raise our hands and look around nervously. I see a harmless-looking man in a check shirt and move over to him. 'Would you like to OM?' he says, using the required words. 'Yes, I would. I have a number one but if you'd like to be my two that would be perfect.'

T finds a number two woman. She smiles at me. I smile back. T comes over to check out the man who has found me. 'Don't worry. I'll take care of your woman,' he says graciously. Hearing me referred to as his woman, T looks comforted.

'You will be my first ever OM Circle partner other than my regular partner,' I say to him. 'It's an honour,' he replies. T is happier.

'So if you could move to your places for the first OM now?' says the woman leading. Everyone else is settled.

'There's a spare place over there.' T and I crossed the

room nervously. No one is paying the least attention to the two newbies. Each couple is focusing on themselves.

I lie down on a mat with T. We're both too hyped up to relax.

'Damn, too much lube,' T says. 'Sorry.'

I laugh. There is a woman next to me moaning gently with pleasure. Oh, heavens, isn't this the experience that I'm supposed to be having? She's obviously more open than I am. 'Comparison is the thief of joy, Isabel,' I tell myself. Then I wonder who said that, was it Theodore Roosevelt or Franklin Roosevelt? Do I have my Roosevelts muddled up? Or was it Franklin's wife, Eleanor Roosevelt? Wouldn't it be more likely to have been her? She's the amazing woman who said, 'No one can patronize you without your consent.' Learnt that one years ago. It's rumoured he had a lover. It's also rumoured that she did too and that they both knew and were happy with this arrangement. How interesting that they are known for those quotes. Maybe he used to patronise her and she compared herself to him and knew that this made her unhappy. Maybe she'd have been the better politician. Then I realize that five minutes has gone by and I'm completely in my head.

I become aware of more gently quiet moaning from another corner of the room. But mostly the room is quiet. Thank God for that. No demonstrations of ability to climax here. No one seems to be noticing anyone else's process anyway. What is T doing? Come on Isabel, take some responsibility here, give an instruction.

'That feels like good pressure, could you try a slightly

different position?' It always takes all my courage giving these gentle instructions.

'Yes. Totally distracted. Sorry,' says T.

'Me too.' I didn't admit that I'd been thinking about possible dynamics in the Roosevelts' marriage.

We have both lost anything that we learnt from our private lesson. It's a disaster. The first OM ends. T and I are both too overwhelmed to be able to focus.

We are supposed to describe a sensation we each experienced during the OM but we just hug.

'If the men could now move into place for the second OM,' says a voice.

My rather charming man arrives. 'I'm a bit nervous,' I admit.

'Don't worry,' he says. 'So am I. I've only just done the training.' Oh heck, I have a beginner. I lie there and actually the humour of the situation overtakes me. Normally I am nervous about giving instructions because somehow it's about me. I allow my inhibitions and my co-dependent desire to look after someone else's feelings to get in the way of my ability to give clear instructions. But now my fears desert me because this man needs help. I have to give instructions. He's clueless.

'That feels good and could you move a little and see if you can see the clitoris at all?'

'Ah,' he says.

'Yes, that's closer.' (Say something positive first.) 'Now, if you move a little closer to the centre?'

'OK.'

'That's a better position. Now, in terms of pressure, if you could try using the tip of your finger rather than the pad? I think you are using the pad?'

'Yes.'

'Could you try a light, short stroke using the tip?'

Suddenly all my inhibitions have gone. I'm a feedback machine.

'Thank you,' he says. 'These instructions are very helpful.'

He keeps going but he hasn't established contact or isn't yet aware that it's possible to. He has my full attention but for the wrong reason. I'm thinking, 'How do I direct him now? He's way off. He doesn't seem to know what he's aiming for.' I wonder who he is, whether he has a partner, what's brought him here. Then I try to focus on the sensation but end up focusing on the lack of sensation instead. Then I try not to judge him or myself and just accept what is. It's not as though anything he's doing feels bad. It feels good. I just feel a bit like a cello where someone's only playing one string rather tentatively. It was very endearing though. Very gentle. Perhaps it was perfect.

The 15 minutes ends. We thank each other rather bashfully and he disappears into the night. T appears. 'How was it?' I ask.

'It was very different from you. She was a very different shape; I found it hard to find her clit. How was it for you?'

'He was a beginner. All my fear of giving feedback was gone and I found I was able to give some directions.'

'Oh.'

'But T. He doesn't stroke as well as you do.'

Some part of T needs to hear this I think.
I take him by the arm. 'Can we go and eat now?' I ask.
'Yes, and can we go home and have sex after that?'
This is called 'asking for what you want'. We're learning.

• • •

It's amazing how one adjusts. If someone had told me a year ago that I would be doing this on a Wednesday evening I wouldn't have believed them. Last night T and I went to the OM Circle in East London. About 25 people gathering in the upstairs of a church building. I wonder if the clergy have any idea what we are doing in their sacred space? Of course I would argue that what we are doing is completely honouring to God – if there is a God. A part of a woman's body exists which has no other purpose than to give the woman pleasure. Yet there are women everywhere that never have this part of their body touched and there are unhappy and frustrated men that would love to touch this part of a woman's body and learn how to give pleasure – but never have the opportunity. Then there are the men that are married and whose wives go cold on them because they never experience pleasure, not because the man wants to withhold anything but because he simply has no idea how to create it. He's probably worrying that his penis isn't hard enough. So which world is crazy? This one, where men are learning and women are teaching them and receiving pleasure at the same time – or the more 'normal' bedrooms which may, or may not, be filled with pleasure?

We walk in for the weekly practice. Men are laying out

mats. 'Hello – my name's Mary – what's yours?' A friendly smiling face greets me. 'Isabel ...' I say. She looks so sane. 'Have you been doing this long? I mean, coming here on a Wednesday night?'

'I've been practising for about three months.' She smiles. 'Yes, it's weird isn't it? It's amazing how quickly it becomes normal.'

Nothing feels 'normal' yet for T or me. The evening contains two 15-minute OMs. Some couples practise exclusively with their partners. But the majority are OMing with different people to learn.

'How many of the people here are single, Mary?' I ask, looking around at a room of men who were, it has to be said, of above-average good looks.

'Some are, some are married, and some are in polyamorous relationships.'

Polyamorous relationships? Oh, good grief.

One Wednesday evening, Rachel – who now runs the Europe branch of OneTaste – asks me casually, 'Would you like to OM?'

OH MY GOD!

Would I like to have a woman stroke my clitoris? Everything in me screams 'NO!' Can I just run away now?

The week this happened T was away and I was there alone for the first time. I'm so straight I'm boring. My skin is very happy next to a man's skin and I've never had any particular desire to put any of it next to a woman's. But there is something about the OM practice that is strangely un-sexual. Although it certainly sounds sexual doesn't it?

A woman stroking your clitoris?

Here they are so matter of fact about it. They do this practice every day, and so my reasons to say, 'No, thank you,' would be what? Fear? Of what exactly? I teach that exploring what makes you afraid is expansive. Am I to be one of those people who doesn't practise what I preach? Sheesh, I'm not bored. I'm as way outside any zone of comfort as I could imagine. Yet perfectly safe in the container of a room full of OM practitioners.

'I'm a very experienced stroker,' she adds – as a masseuse might if they saw you hesitate before accepting a shoulder massage. There's no hook. It isn't a come-on. She's straight and wants nothing – except maybe to demonstrate to me some sensation that I may not have had before ... to follow the musical analogy – some new notes.

The only reason to say 'no' would be fear, conditioning and habitual preference. A reason to say 'yes' is that it may enrich my practice and, once again, teach me. I'm not sure how T would feel about it but he's on holiday. The choice is mine. I take a deep breath. 'OK, Rachel.' I can't believe I just said that. I really can't.

'And how was it?' I hear you asking. Well, it was different. Rachel managed 'grindy' and 'intense' and 'gentle' all in the same OM. And she certainly hit some notes that I hadn't experienced before. Notes of a different pitch that made me feel like a different instrument. But sheesh – I'll be very glad to go back to men at the next OM Circle. Men will always be my preference. I'm just made that way.

In the sharing afterwards I blush. 'I just had my first-ever

OM with a woman. I can't believe I did that.'

Twenty-five people applaud. Another boundary bites the dust. I'm learning to be a little more open. I guess this is all part of this journey. I notice that the world goes on turning just the same but maybe I just became one fraction less inhibited than I was yesterday, one fraction less narrow-minded even. Sheesh, this is hard.

Orgasmic Meditation Training Day – with Live Demonstration

Meanwhile I haven't forgotten tantra or other aspects of my sexuality. And I'm still reading.

The last truly comprehensive study of female orgasm was in the Masters and Johnson classics from 1966 and 1970. Both these concluded that penile thrusting during intercourse should be enough to bring a woman to orgasm. Shere Hite's *Report on Female Sexuality* in 1976 told us that only 33% of women reached orgasm through intercourse alone. So, was it their conclusion that there was something wrong with all the rest of us? Yes – somehow that was implied. No one, even now, seems to make it really clear that male and female response is very different. It throws me into a little rage. As recently as 1998, an Australian urologist, Helen O'Connell, wrote that the unerect clitoris (which is mostly internal) can be up to nine centimetres long and yet is considered co-incidental by many men as the centre for women's sexual pleasure. In 2013 the artist

Sophia Wallace started her 'Cliteracy' campaign, and slogans started to appear in New York street art and dotted across Facebook and Twitter that said things like, 'A man would never be expected to get off through sex acts that ignored his primary sexual organ.'[13] And 'Terrorism is having sex your entire adult life, giving birth to six children and never experiencing an orgasm.' But Sophia wasn't blaming men – women also have to take some responsibility for this with a slogan, 'Tell the truth. Women will never be equal to men so long as they are having bad sex and lying about it.' The message is clear – the reality out there is dire – both for men and for women and the only thing I can do is keep going. Keep taking responsibility.

The OM community does workshops. One-day workshops where they teach groups of people how to OM. Nicole comes to London about twice a year and runs them. T tells me, 'They do a live demonstration of the OM.'

'They do what?'

'On stage. A woman lies on stage and Nicole demonstrates. As part of the workshop. Then in the afternoon they teach and then they end the day and anyone who wants to can stay and OM.'

'These things happen in London?'

T and I want to learn. We cancel everything and sign up. It's only a day after all. The workshop is at London's beautiful Asia House which makes me smile. The last time I'd been there was to hear William Dalrymple. This is a little different. I think William would enjoy it.

• • •

Nicole is punctual and dressed, quite consciously, in a drop-dead gorgeous figure-hugging red dress that screams 'sex' at all the men in the audience. I swear she sits on a high stool to present with her legs ever so slightly apart quite deliberately. This event is called 'Turn On' and she makes sure that the day lives up to expectations.

'Is she wearing anything under that dress?' I whisper to T.

'There is no visible panty line. Not that I've looked. Of course.'

Then Nicole starts to speak in a mixture of stand-up comedy, motivational talk, neuro-linguistic programming and sex lecture rolled into one. She's funny and my pen can't write fast enough to take all the notes I want.

'When I first started the OM practice I basically cried for three years.'

Hmm, she has to be exaggerating right? But saying this gives permission to all the women that get emotional during the practice – which I don't. She says in the book that for the first six months she didn't feel anything at all. So we learn that if I, or any other women, feel very little, we know not to worry.

Then, in a seamless flow, she says to the men, 'If a woman is not turned on you can do no right. You can be stroking with the utmost precision and nothing will happen. If she is turned on, touch her knee and she'll love it.'

So now all the men would be feeling better. I scribble notes furiously.

'I've never seen anyone who is beyond redemption,' she says. Hooray. Listen to that, Mr Freud. Listen to that everyone who has been sexually abused or knows anyone who has been. Listen to that any woman who has some kind of sexual problem. I think of a woman I know who has vaginismus, and others who experience pain on penetration or who are frustrated because they simply don't like sex. In saying 'no' to bad sex they have thrown away pleasure too.

'I've never seen anyone who is beyond redemption.' I write the words in my notebook in block capitals. Good for Nicole.

'Women, we want men who are strong but also somehow intuitively able to read our minds. When men can't see a way to move forward then their minds go into paralysis and then we complain that our men are not engaged.'

Yes – women I know complain that their men are checked out.

'Don't apply the rules of production to orgasm. It requires a lot more feeling around in the dark than having a formula. It's nuanced; a state of nuance in which all of you is required. Orgasm is an involuntary state. It's about flow. Flow isn't self-conscious.'

She jumps around – deliberately I'm sure – from subject to subject. It's more like entertainment than a lecture.

'Play around with yearning. Play with tension in the body. Don't have sex with her, men, until it's irresistible. Give her a chance to show off for you in bed. Play with power dynamics that you are not normally comfortable with. Break rules in the bedroom. You are consenting adults and you may discover unbelievable pleasure when you break the rules. No one wants sex that is reliable, punctual sex.'

Ha ha ha. Punctual sex. Oh dear. I remember a friend who complained to me that she felt her man scheduled in the sex, in the diary, along with his other obligations.

'And don't be "nice",' she said. 'We can nice each other to death.' Hmm, T and I are nice to each other. Perhaps too nice.

'You need a little dissonance in the relationship,' Nicole advises. 'Experiment. If you're in a cosy relationship, try doing something deliberately to piss the other one off. You'll discover that a little dissonance has advantages.'

I have heard this before – couples that tell me those rows are good for their sex lives. I'm convinced that it's not necessary and not very enlightened. On the other hand, couples that never row can end up not communicating honestly or in depth. Can you disagree fiercely and not row? And if you don't row, can you still have 'dissonance'? Hmmm. Discuss.

Then she talks about 'vigilance', one of the keys to women having a good sexual experience.

'Your brain's vigilance centre is like a meerkat on a mound looking all around and screaming.' Both the man and the woman have to calm down the vigilance centres so that you can be completely focused on sensations. Once the vigilance centre is relaxed you can explore the ten different spots on the clitoris and the natural point of highest sensitivity, which, as you now know, is the upper left hand quadrant.

'The 8,000 nerve endings there begin to unwind and the sensation is enough to draw you out of your personal narrative.'

Only sometimes, I say to myself.

'And then the spot that no one can find – grows.'

Oh, I hope so.

Then she describes the possible feeling that comes from four different types of stroke. T and I haven't explored this so I'm paying attention.

'A very fast stroke creates a feeling of reverence and of reaching out. An upstroke feels like rising – literally like going up – like a balloon. A downstroke is the exhale – it can feel low and kind of gritty. Stroking the back of the clit makes the strokee feel, "Oh, I love you. I'll do anything for you." And how does the stroker learn to play to get a pitch-perfect response?'

Good question.

'It's to do with watching the channels of feedback. Don't trust the sounds that she makes, as women are prone either to exaggerating with sound or they don't give any feedback at all. It can be difficult for the woman being stroked. I remember when I started I couldn't say whether I was receiving an upstroke or a downstroke and everything felt as though the sensation was more in the reservoir on the left than on the clit itself.'

'So how does the man tell what's really a good sensation and what isn't if she isn't giving clear feedback?' a young man asked, pen in hand.

'That's why you have your right thumb at the base of the introitus, just slightly inside so that you can feel muscle contractions. Also, if you have a good stroke she will produce more liquid, which is involuntary and can't be faked. Those are your guides.'

Very good.

'It sounds difficult and there's a lot to learn,' complains a man in the front row.

'Don't forget that it's a goal-less practice. For the woman the only goal is to feel every stroke. For the stroker all you have to do is make your finger feel good.'

'So it's easy?' asks a young woman. The audience is totally engaged.

'It's as easy as meditation where all you do is focus on the breath. It takes a second to learn but many people have spent years in caves focusing on the breath so there must be some benefit.'

'I don't get it. I thought this was about how to have an orgasm?' asks a woman.

'What you are calling orgasm we call "climax". I like to sneeze too but it's really not what we are after here. We are going for an experience that is much deeper, much longer and there is no comparison. But you don't have to take my word for it. We invite you to give it a go.'

'Are you constantly thinking about sex, Nicole?' asks an attractive older man.

She laughs.

'No, I'm constantly thinking about sensation.'

'What about masturbation? Can't you do this for yourself?' asks a man rather charmingly.

'No. Masturbation increases your vigilance centre. You can't relax completely and be in control of yourself. But someone else can. We have this need for another person programmed into us.' That's why it feels so much better when someone else does it, because we can relax more.

There's something very inviting in all these words. Later I found that I had written in my notebook, 'There is a space in me for what you are saying.' But when I read it I didn't know whether it was something that Nicole had said to the person who introduced this to her, or whether it was something I'd said. It summed up what I felt pretty well.

What Nicole is offering, and with huge positive energy, is possibility. Somehow it's a way forward that's honest. Not easy, but honest and requiring a new kind of courage. It feels like wide space opening up, a new horizon; new possibilities. And I feel proud. Proud of them for the new hope they are bringing to so many couples and the new hope of intimacy and connection for those that aren't in couples. Proud for the fact that they have come from the US to teach us inhibited Brits to ask for what we want a bit more. Proud that this audience is sitting here, outside the social norms. After all, where have the social norms got us? Divorce – one in three? Or is it one in two these days? Happy marriages? Happy people? Sexually blissed-out and loved-up couples? Not a lot of it about is there? So I'm proud that we're in the room.

And for you too. And I'm proud of you – still reading. Still exploring.

• • •

Now it's the demonstration. I'm scared that they'll have a close-up camera that will show all-singing all-dancing vagina muscles vibrating with pleasure – the Olympic Gold Medal for fitness and mega-skilled pussy that would show mine up to be more like a floppy old pair of slippers. I'm scared of her experience too – that she'll have a massive climax after about seven minutes and another one after the next three and I'll be scarred for life by the trauma of watching. I'll have nightmares in which I'll see her muscles, forever in close up, taunting me with their brilliance. And T was similarly scared that after watching what could be done he would feel inadequate and unworthy to be allowed anywhere near one of these astounding miracles of the natural world.

We're certainly both nervous.

'No. I was excited,' says T later. OK. So, I'm nervous and T is excited.

There's no close-up camera. But we're in the second row so we have a completely clear view.

The room starts to fill with an almost electric energy before they begin. The excitement is welcome but the comparisons are not. Nicole diffuses that part of the experience before she starts. 'Now, before we do the demo I'm going to give you the rules. There is only one rule, OK? You are not allowed to judge yourselves during the OM. This is an incremental process and we have both being doing this a long time and have become more and more free. Even if you are OMing now no one would expect you to be at this level. So you have to promise not to compare and judge yourselves, OK? If you don't promise I won't let you stay,' Nicole jokes. We raise our hands and promise not to judge ourselves. No eternal scarring for me then.

'You can't OM wrong but you can OM with greater

resonance and there is a point where giving and receiving become one.'

To go back to the analogy of a musician, we're about to watch a concert standard performance. Nicole is a player of the clitoris who has been playing every day for 20 years and has played, as she said, thousands of different instruments.

'This is just to show you what is possible. It's not for you to compare. It's for your inspiration.'

If everyone who saw a master cellist decided that they may as well give up as they'd never be able to play that well – we'd have very few good musicians. Most musicians watch a maestro and go home to practise. Or, in this case, be practised on.

The room buzzes with nervous tension. It feels as you'd feel before an important date or a job interview for a job that you really want, people are barely breathing and we aren't even participating – we're just watching.

Then Justine comes forward. Oh my God – Justine is the woman who's going to get on to the table and be played by Nicole? Sweet, lovely, warm Justine who had been so kind when T and I went for our private session. What courage. On the other hand, I suppose she is the head of 'Turn On UK' (the UK part of OneTaste) so she has to lead by example. But still … I hold my breath for her even though she seems completely relaxed.

She takes off her underwear, climbs on the table and butterflies her legs so that all the room can see. I'm guessing that this was the first time that many people had seen between a woman's legs for some years, or ever. Nicole explains in an almost medical way what she's going to do. 'I measure what I'm doing by the involuntary contractions of the introitus. I never trust the sounds a woman makes. I hear them but I don't allow them to guide me.' Then she turns to Justine.

'Are you OK?'

Justine's completely OK. She's completely calm. I guess this isn't the first demo that she's ever done in front of a large audience.

Nicole takes off her heels and puts on the super-fine gloves. I know how super-fine as my number two man at the OM Circle wore them and I couldn't feel them.

Nicole asks the audience, 'During the OM if you could call out any sensations you are feeling, it helps release them into the room.' Someone says 'tense tummy' before she starts.

'Please breathe.'

She explains how much lube to use:

'About a dime-sized amount on your left index finger so that it doesn't run out – and if it does for some reason, get more; even if it's in the middle of stroking, and just let your partner know. With the "OneTaste" lube, it's very easy to use and isn't runny. If you use liquid lube it'll get messy.'

She puts some lube on her stroking finger – and then starts to play. As she plays she tells us about the strokes that she's using. I can't take notes. I just sit in amazement, as we all do, with our pulses racing.

'I'm going to go straight in with quite a firm stroke at the beginning to establish the connection.' It's really like watching Yo-Yo Ma sweeping down with his bow and hearing the cello sing. Justine started to make noises like a well-tuned cello. I don't mean the kind of over-the-top screaming that you hear in low-rate porn or sex on TV – I mean soft, low groans that come from some deep place in her.

'Then a very light stroke increases the sensation.' Nicole is utterly focused and connected with Justine but also aware of the room. Justine's breathing changes and she starts to make a different kind of music. Powerful stuff. Everyone in the room is aroused in some way or other. Men and women – with a mixture of shock, admiration and awe.

'And the upstroke takes her higher.' Justine starts to gasp and pant. We all start to. The notes that are coming out of Justine also get higher. She grasps the bed and then lets go again. I seem to sense the sensation rise in her.

'A downstroke gives a grindy, earthy sensation.' Nicole says. As we are near the front we can see her finger moving really quite fast. Far faster than T has ever played me. She is certainly confident in her playing. Justine's making a different sound – deeper, much more grounded.

'And it feels good to see how deep you can take someone, as well as how high.'

Nicole's smiling as she both creates and shares the pleasure. I want to laugh. It's not nerves, it's the sheer undiluted joy in Nicole. I've seen Yo-Yo Ma play the cello too. It's the same kind of pure exhilaration – only better as very few people as far as I'm aware experience the kind of pleasure when watching Yo-Yo Ma that the audience is feeling here today.

'Then, when you go behind the clit that is a different

sensation again,' I remember earlier that Nicole had said this is the sensation that makes the strokee want to declare undying love to the stroker. I didn't see Justine about to do that but from the sounds that she was making we could get an impression of the experience that she was having.

Nicole speaks to the person right at the middle of the front row who is almost immediately between Justine's legs. 'Look carefully at the muscular contractions – those are involuntary and they are my guide as well as what I feel. Anyone else who wants to come forward and look, go ahead.'

This may seem to you to be a little unfair on Justine to have half the room invited to come and look between her legs but Justine was very happy in that moment. Believe me.

'Then when you've taken a woman way down you can take her way up again.'

We almost feel the metaphorical sweep of the bow as Nicole changes strokes.

'Will everyone in the room please exhale?' Nicole smiles. 'You are all part of this experience. Justine is in a state of heightened sensitivity right now and feels everything in the room. It's hard to her to relax fully if you all stop breathing.' We breathe out obediently.

'Then when she's up there you can just let her fly for a while if you maintain it with a light stroke.' By this time everyone who had started nervous and tense has relaxed and is enjoying the ride.

'Who would like to come forward and feel the energy?' Nicole asks. A few brave souls raise their hand. 'Come then.' Another well-dressed helper with a name badge that says

'Rachel' directs people to come forward and very gently lay their hands on Justine's thighs. Both men and women come forward. I raise my hand and am invited forward. I lay my hands very gently on Justine's upper thigh and can feel, quite clearly, a form of electricity run through me. The same that I feel if I am pleasuring T. But here I'm just standing fully clothed in a room of a hundred people. I notice the subtlety and the strength of the sensation that travels into my hands and up my arms, passes through me and warms my head and my toes. After perhaps a minute Rachel makes a signal for me to step back and for the next person to step forward. T raises his hand and takes a turn and all this time Nicole, standing on the other side of Justine, plays on lightly – just keeping her at a very high point of vibration ... or something. Thirteen minutes and Nicole says – 'OK, I'm just going to spend the last two minutes grounding her – bringing her back down to earth.' The sounds coming out of Justine change again. We watch and listen. My heart is pumping with admiration. 'And lower,' Nicole says. 'And I just press on her pelvic bone at the end to make sure that all that energy goes into her and can be used. Men you'll be surprised how hard you can press at this point. Strokee, if your stroker doesn't press hard enough during this last grounding then just grab his arm yourself and pull it down to help him.'

You could hear a pin drop in the room.

'And that's time.'

Justine sits up, looks at the room with a huge, pure, natural blissed-out smile. The room breaks into generous applause. For Nicole, for the amazing playing and for

Justine, for the sheer undiluted generosity and guts of what she has just done. Some people in the room are laughing and some are crying. We give them a standing ovation. The audience would be cheering too but we're too dumbfounded.

'Well T, if I've seen anything more extraordinary than that in my life, I can't remember what it was.'

'That was it for me.'

You too can see this. You can't say that I don't introduce some interesting possibilities for Saturdays out in London, right?

• • •

In the afternoon Nicole has gone and another bouncy, sexy American woman in a slightly less red dress takes over. She explains how to OM by giving all the men a pencil with a little rubber on top and showing how best to stroke it.

Then there is a simple exercise where you walk around the room and ask, 'Would you like to OM?' and receive the reply 'yes' or 'no'. Then they repeat it so someone asks you, 'Would you like to OM?' And you reply either 'yes' or 'no'. With all options open the practical part of the day begins for all those that want to stay and experience OM. For most of these brave souls it will be the first time.

Very few people leave. Maybe ten. The rest, those who have come to this event alone, are about to walk up to a total stranger and say, 'Would you like to OM?' There are women who are able to do this? I definitely wouldn't have the courage to be here if I didn't have T at my side.

While we've been out for the break they've built 'nests'.

We have our own cushions, towels and scarves that we've brought. Opposite our little nest, a woman in a wheelchair is being helped onto a table by two men. Surely she isn't here alone?

'Did you just choose a partner from the room?' I ask her.

'No,' she smiles, 'this is my husband.' I'm relieved. This is hard enough without the vulnerability of having to ask a stranger to remove your underwear and spread your legs for you.

The OM starts. I'm more nervous than usual but T's been inspired by the demo and wants to make use of what he's seen. He uses a faster stroke than he has done before and I notice what a different sensation it produces. A bit like finding a new note that he's never played before. Rachel walks around to each couple giving an instruction or two. When she reaches us she says to T. 'Stroke with intention. Penetrate her with your stroke.'

'What?' said T, momentarily distracted from his playing.

Penetrate with the stroke? What does that mean? Does it just mean stroke more firmly? Or if it means to stroke with a clearer intention – just exactly what is the intention in a goal-less OM? There are so many levels to this amazing practice.

I go back to enjoying the sensation – and the experimentation. Both experiencing the beginnings of new tunes, new notes, new rhythms, and the anticipation of what notes these could become when we are braver. This is courage of a different kind. There is so much mystery in our bodies.

The 15 minutes ends (always a sad moment) and T and I sit

and hug each other. Overwhelmed by the close proximity of others, overwhelmed by the day, overwhelmed by everything.

I managed to ask Justine a quick question:

'About the different strokes?'

'Ah, the spots on the clit and the strokes … Yes. They are difficult to talk about because people tend to leap to concretizing them and the clitoris doesn't work like that. In general, though, a fast light stroke at the 1 o'clock spot has a feeling of reverence. Stroking the 6 o'clock spot quite firmly is like fucking and a stroke of the 3 o'clock spot is like love.'

I had experienced none of these differences. T and I had mainly been experimenting with a medium stroke at 1 o'clock as the book instructed.

'But …' Justine continued.

'Here is the hard part – none of this is created by the stroker. It can only be evoked if present between the stroker and strokee.'

Then why are we being encouraged to OM with strangers with whom we may not have any chemistry? But Justine was gone. So many people want her attention. Imagine running a community based on sexuality. Brave woman.

There is one final exercise. We all gather in one room and sit in a circle. Everyone is asked to speak out one or a few words about their experience.

There are many of us so I don't write anything down. I have no idea what T and I said. There is just one response that stands out in my mind. A man, laughing, says, 'What exactly have I been doing in my life until today?'

Late Summer Adventure

So now, assuming you are still reading, we are going on an adventure. I've been invited to visit San Francisco to attend a conference as a guest of Nicole Daedone and the OneTaste Community. I've never been to the West Coast of America, let alone to attend a conference about sexuality and clitoral stroking. I thought you may be curious to know what would happen. T can't come and he's hugely disappointed and boiling with envy. But all I need is my notebook and I can take you along. No expensive tickets necessary. Just make sure you're sitting comfortably.

The First International Conference of
Clitoris Stroking

This morning I woke up in San Francisco. The sun is shining and I'm experiencing the now familiar feeling of mild terror.

This is day one of 'OMX – the Orgasmic Meditation Experience'. And it's the first international conference primarily about clitoris stroking (weirder and weirder) and somehow I'm here. There are lectures from leading experts on female sexuality but it isn't just academic, it's hands on. Obviously.

There are over 1,000 people here in a good gender balance, and in one very large room 500 'nests' have been set up. As if that isn't challenging enough I'm also staying at the San Francisco OM community where 50 of those who practice this extraordinary form of human connection live together.

Every morning at 7.30 they have an OM Circle as their morning practice. They do one orgasmic meditation with one partner for 15 minutes and then a second for 15 minutes, usually with another partner.

I'm able to walk up to any man here and say, 'Would you like to OM?' and he will say either 'yes' or 'no'. In my experience men rarely say 'no' unless they have practical reasons, in which case they'll say, 'I'm not sure when we could.' Or, 'I'd love to but ...' Mostly they say, 'Yes. When?' especially with any new partner.

You may be thinking, 'Isabel, have you lost your mind and your soul? Aren't you the person who wrote about Tibet? Who interviewed His Holiness the Dalai Lama? The Isabel who cares about spirituality? Morality? Ethics? Love?' Yes, this is still me. Please keep reading.

You see, I have a simple and staggeringly obvious observation from many years of study, about the current rules system in our society. It simply doesn't work, does it? I'm not suggesting that we should run away from marriage and monogamy – of course not. But I am suggesting that – based on the current divorce rates, the additional number of people that are not divorced but are having affairs, the couples that are neither divorced nor having affairs but are simply not happy in their bedrooms – based on the sum total of human unhappiness and loneliness I see in relationships around me, I think it's worth examining our conditioning and the status quo.

What I hate about the current system is the lies. It seems that to lie is necessary for far too many people. People lie to protect their partners from the truth and worse – they lie to themselves and pretend that they are happy in a relationship when they may be screaming for freedom. It seems that relatively few of us can make it work.

I'm also not saying that living in a community based on a particular consensual sexual practice is any more likely to succeed in the long run. I'm just saying that, based on the statistics, it's good for us to consider other models in case we can learn something. OK?

There is kindness and generosity here. Both men and women 'OM' with people who, in our 'normal' society wouldn't stand a chance of getting any sexual needs met – or even any simple human connection. You see young women say 'yes' to an OM request from men that, frankly, I find repulsive. And I see beautiful men OM with women who are three times their age or three times their size. Similarly: class, race, career status, religion, politics – none of these thing matter here. 'Would you like to OM?' Answer: 'Yes, please.' Or, 'No, thank you.' If someone says, 'No, thank you,' ask someone else. The lack of a feeling of scarcity is very unusual.

Those who are more experienced practise OM with a far wider range of partners than I would ever be capable of having such a connection with. It's hard not to have preferences. Some of the leaders in this community have had years of Buddhist experience. Buddhism teaches us to have neither 'attraction' nor 'aversion' and this is certainly a place to realize the clarity of that. The greatest challenge, for me, is not asking for an OM, which some find hard, nor a fear of rejection – if a man says 'no', that's his prerogative – the problem is finding men I want to ask.

But I'm here and feeling very alive. I'm looking out for men I feel comfortable to approach. I try to read them on an energetic level. Does this sound unlikely to you? Me looking at a room of men wondering which ones I'd like to ask? It sounds unlikely to me too. I guess I've come a long way since I wrote that first letter to T and was terrified even to OM with him. It seems that it is possible for us to learn slowly, to drop some of our inhibitions.

I've now relaxed a bit and asked several men here if they'd like an OM partner at some point in the conference and they've all said 'yes.' It's a bit like going to an old-fashioned dance where you learn that you need ten dance partners and you only have two lined up.

It's 11am as I write this. The conference starts in an hour. How am I feeling? Nervous. And how is my clitoris feeling? Well, as they say around these parts, 'Like – totally awesome.'

• • •

Five hundred nests with 500 couples and we all OM at the same time. Many women seem to love this experience. They say that they can feel the energy of the room and it enhances their sensation. I heard one woman in the queue going in saying, 'I'm so excited I can barely breathe.' Some people are moved to tears, some are laughing and, and ...

I hate this. There's a woman about two nests from me who is making weirdly loud retching and groaning sounds during the OM. I'm concerned that she's about to be sick. An assistant approaches and tells her to relax and breathe.

I'm thinking of the cup of coffee I'm going to treat myself to when the OM ends. It's interesting to notice though that when my mind is elsewhere I feel almost nothing. I suppose if I was a little more advanced in my practice I'd say, 'I'm sorry, can you stop please? I can't do this with a woman sounding tortured beside us and I feel far too distracted to feel any sensation at all.' This is a practice based on pleasure and if I don't tell the poor man that I'm having a bad time and not feeling any pleasant sensation how is he going to know? Not that I've ever done anything remotely similar to this during actual sex. Of course. Not.

• • •

So now, with coffee, I'm sitting in a large auditorium and they are pumping out music with a loud bass – Anthony Robbins-style hype. This is so far from the subtle beauty of the clitoral strokes that we are here to learn how to give and receive. Am I at the wrong event?

'We are here to celebrate orgasm!' a young woman leads from the stage. Everyone cheers. 'One thousand three hundred people registered!' everyone cheers. They list the countries and cities, 'And who is here from Las Vegas??' A small group shouts. 'I said, 'Who is here from Las Vegas???' They obligingly cheer louder. 'And who is here from New

York?' More obliging cheers – and so on. Then amusingly she says, 'Who is here from the EU? Total silence. I've met people from France, Germany, Ireland, Spain and Holland, but no one thinks of themselves as 'from the EU!' so this is met by silence. Then the crowd whipper-upper starts on – 'And who has been OMing for a long time?' We cheer. 'And who is new to OMing?' We cheer. They dance and say, 'That's AWESOME!!' a lot. I understand that they want to celebrate. It's taken work to get 'OneTaste' to their first international event and I'm being grumpy. They'd say I'm not 'turned on'. They'd be right.

Finally, at 8pm, Nicole comes on and starts to talk sense and I relax and enjoy her as always. She tells us that millions of women in the US take medication because they have a new condition – 'Female sexual arousal disorder.' I have no idea whether this is supposed to be an actual figure that she's giving us but there are certainly 'a lot of' women' taking medication. None of the women here are: that's for certain.

I look it up later. This 'condition' is defined as 'the inability to attain or maintain sexual arousal'. It's further defined as the 'inability to maintain arousal until the completion of a sexual activity'. Hmmm. What do you suppose they mean by that? Is it possible that they are defining having a climax as the 'completion of the sexual activity?' And if women don't 'maintain arousal', are they now sick? I wonder, does the doctor stop to ask any questions before this diagnosis? Does he know where your clitoris is? Do you know where your clitoris is? Do you like each other at all?

It gets worse. We can also now be diagnosed with

'hypoactive sexual desire disorder'. This one is characterized by a 'lack or absence of sexual fantasies and desire for sexual activity for some period of time.' So, if we are not enjoying sexual fantasies, we now need medicating? Do you suppose that there is the least chance that this is because someone is expecting a woman's mind to work like a man's? And what do they mean by 'fantasies' exactly?

So, all you celibate people or all you people that are not actively having fantasies – you are sick. Rush to the doctor and say, 'I think I'm suffering from hypoactive sexual desire disorder.' Or if your sexual desire drops off during your sexual activity, regardless of the reason, that makes you sick too. I don't think so. Don't people love to tell us that we need drugs?

The reason that Nicole is also passionate about this is that with the OM practice – where the man is actually learning – in the greatest and most subtle detail – how to give a woman pleasure ... what do we find? Well, with a little training of the man and patience, 100% of women who have a clitoris can learn to receive pleasure during an OM.

Nicole believes that orgasm needs to be a practice – just as yoga is a practice for the body and meditation is a practice for the mind. We can learn to receive pleasure. Nicole is speaking to us in visionary terms of the possibility of a different status quo.

'How would it be if we lived in a world where being appropriate is not considered better than being honest?'

'How would it be if we simply let the small animal of our body love what it loves?' she said, quoting the wonderful poem 'Wild Geese' by Mary Oliver.[14]

'How would it be to live in an OM-based world where we all had as much experience of orgasmic energy as we wanted?'

Nicole tells us about the pleasure that men find in learning this and of the pleasure that they learn to feel through the woman's arousal. She uses the phrase 'the honey blanket'. How glorious.

Nicole has a vision of a world where this kind of connection is available to all – just as yoga and meditation is. She would like to see the three practices coming naturally together in people's minds and diaries. There are no conditions for entry. You don't need to be relatively fit as you do to enjoy yoga or even able to sit still as you need to if you want to enjoy meditation. With OM you just need willingness to learn.

'I want to welcome all of each of you,' she says.

Then, for the newcomers that don't understand what all this is about, Nicole and Justine do a demo with Justine OMing on a platform in front of 1,000 people. It should be remarkable and obviously, for those who are seeing this the first time, it is. But for me somehow putting it on such a huge stage makes it seem like a theatrical event.

I'm confused, bewildered and grumpy so I take a cab back to 1080, the name of the OM house in San Fran that they name by the number of the street. The wonder of living in a community is that there is always someone that you can sit and have a chat with. Sure enough, one of the more elderly residents is sitting there so I make two cups of tea, sit with him and confide in him about my retching neighbour during the group OM and my inability to concentrate.

'It's just like meditation' he says, 'Whatever happens around you – you just bring your awareness back to sensation.'

'Yes. I know the theory. I'm just really not good at it. But in breathing meditation, if I hear roadworks, I know to bring my attention back to the breath.'

'It's the same. Sensation. Not thought.'

'So, I had the best teacher out of all the 500 couples right next to me?'

'You did.'

Pah. Humbug.

'Did you enjoy today?'

'Parts of it. But I compared myself with other women who, based on the sounds they were making, appeared to have greater sensation – and I found myself wanting.'

'I see. We learn not to compare. Even one OM with the next. Even if you have a really resonant OM with one partner it may be flat the next day so we don't compare.'

'I'm not there yet. I'm still judging myself harshly.'

'So did anything really reach you?'

'Yes. There was something Nicole said: that "Oxytocin flows like the land of milk and honey." I've felt that. It's a feeling of milk and honey in the body that this OM practice gives easy access to. I want more of that, for me and for everyone I know. And if this practice is one way of leading people there ... and I'm learning about it ... that's enough for me.'

'Very good,' he says. And I walk up to my bedroom,

passing five or six attractive men who I suspect would be very happy to help me in this research. I'd only have to ask and each of them would say 'yes', 'no' or 'maybe'. I'm glad I'm dating T and don't have to think. I go to my room, and sleep like a happy child.

• • •

One of the most extraordinary claims that they are making in this practice is that the limbic areas of the brain, that is those parts that are responsible for attention and emotional connection, are actually trained by OMing.

In the book *The Brain that Changes Itself*, that Nicole mentioned, Dr Norman Doidge writes that the brain has an ability to repair itself and form new neural pathways. This is what they call neuro-plasticity. Practise, in anything, makes perfect or makes progress and improvement. In the OM practice, you have a man who, as many times a week as possible, is focusing 100% of his attention on noticing the results in a woman, when his finger is stroking her clitoris. He is not thinking about his own sexual satisfaction but is encouraged to put all his attention, initially at least, on her. As you'll remember now, he is encouraged not to be distracted by any sounds that she may make, but to observe, in the greatest detail, the movements in her 'pussy'. (Sheesh, these OMers need a new word for the area between a woman's legs.) By giving her body his primary attention he learns about 'ignition' and 'arousal' in a way that can totally bypass a man during sexual intercourse because he is too caught up in his own arousal and, because his sensation can be intense, it's possible for him to have sex and be completely unaware that she may be feeling very little at all.

In an OM a man focuses on her. He will also feel his own sensation but that is, initially, a secondary focus. Now, the man can develop this exquisite ability to focus on a woman's pleasure, allowing his own to take a secondary role until eventually he becomes so attuned to her sensation that he can barely tell where one ends and the other begins.

It's not going to take him that long to notice that if he doesn't have his finger in the correct location she simply isn't going to respond. The clitoris moves; it's elusive. It's different depending on whether it is erect or not, it both extends and seems to retract, it appears to move from side to side and up and down. Now in case you are thinking 'What? It doesn't move.' We are talking about a question of millimetres here – but a millimetre can make a lot of difference from him being on the clit or off it. When he has found the clit he then has to understand different sensations in different areas in order to arouse her and allow her to explore sensation fully. Remember, our fingers are uniquely sensitive.

If he attempts to 'play' the clit, i.e. experiment with more or less pressure or a faster or slower stoke, before he is sure that he has ignition she may be lying there in her head, just wondering how to give him an 'adjustment' and feeling next to nothing. Just as much as a man would if you stroked the skin next to his penis. Nothing is wrong, for a man, in having the skin next to his penis stroked but, for prolonged periods of stroking, it just wouldn't do it for him.

And feeling this spot correctly is a skill that can be learnt.

And, as the man practises, every day, giving his unique and undivided attention to watching his partner's body (or his partners' bodies depending on how many OM partners he has) the theory is that those parts of his brain – the limbic parts – actually grow stronger. Through observation, attention, patience and vigilance – he is developing sexual empathy. He is learning to recognize and relate to how she FEELS. And while he is doing that the woman's main process is just to lie there, enjoy the ride, keep focusing on the pleasure and keep directing him back to the points of sensation that please her best.

Now does all this sound like theory? This is what I'm here to find out. Some of the men here have been practising a long time. They know their instrument and their limbic capacity is developed. I am here to learn from these men and to take what I learn back to my practice with T.

• • •

Saturday morning begins better for me. I search the local streets around the conference centre for a coffee shop that isn't part of a chain where I can have coffee in a cup without plastic, and manage to find one. And I overhear some conference organizers voicing one of my concerns. Which pleases me.

I guess the concern about 'selling' – 'hard selling' and 'soft selling' – must come up in any organization. More so when people really love and care about the product. But you may imagine that where the product is related to a new form of access to the pleasures of human sexuality – feelings run very deep indeed.

A woman in a 'OneTaste' T-shirt isn't happy.

'What is on offer here is no less than a path for women to their own orgasm and a path for men to access this most exquisite connection. We don't need to sell any of our courses actively and it's quite wrong to do so. The product sells itself to those who want it.'

It seems she had heard another staff member selling the 'Mastery' course they offer in a way that had seemed inappropriate to her. She continues,

'There is no need to be even 1% pushy. Anyone can sell this course because if anyone wants this they will ask. We don't have to sell. We just have to offer.'

'Yes,' said the second staff member. 'You don't feel that – on this occasion – this was done?'

'No.'

I was reassured to overhear this conversation. This organization is definitely 'monetized' – to use the American word. This event is hyped and they are selling courses, using all the usual tricks, 'And for the first 15 who sign up ...' blah blah. On the other hand, they have to pay trainers and coaches to fly around the world. They need wages and plane tickets. There is so much that is free – you can have all the whole practice for the price of Nicole's book and who knows how many couples are quietly enjoying OMs without knowing that the community exists? Just as T and I did for months.

The OM Circles are also free. Yoga isn't free. Meditation sometimes is but sometimes meditation courses are expensive. So, just because these people are students of the female orgasm – should they work for free? I think not. Anyway – I was pleased I had heard the discussion. And that someone thought someone else had got it wrong. That's a good sign I think. Healthy debate is good in a community. Also I agreed with her; there was far too much selling going on.

• • •

There is a lot of discussion of desire here. I go to a workshop and am no less clear. It's a complex subject. What do you desire? We move from consideration of purely physical desire – like the force felt by my friend when she smells her boyfriend's skin, to desire in the broadest sense.

I have been reminded that desire, any kind of desire, produces energy. I know that I would walk 500 miles just to see the face of one particular person I know. That's a lot of desire – a lot of energy.

From the point of view of this book and considering what makes sex into the best possible sex, primarily in monogamous relationships, this is a subject worthy of pondering. Even if an animalistic desire exists initially in relationships – how is it to be maintained?

This question brings us to 'attraction'. Attraction is like magnetism. What makes you just want to be close to some people? A man or a woman can exude such good energy that you just want to be close to them. What creates this? Is it happiness with the self? Is it a loving attitude toward others or a rich sense of humour? A sense of someone challenging himself or herself that makes their relationship with life a joyful one? Is it that they have a love of life and an appreciation of all that is? These are the things that make someone attractive to me. The feeling of 'I'd like to be more like this person' is one of the drivers to be close to someone. Isn't it?

None of this is the same as desire. We can find a potential partner that delights us in terms of personality, they may be intelligent and funny and have a list of good qualities but we may have no desire at all to rip their clothes off and get horizontal with them. Someone may appal us but we still want to get naked with them.

For a relationship to work in the long term we have to have both these, don't we? Let's consider attraction first. We have to be attracted to someone not just in the first months where the attraction may be based on projection, but for life. And is this possible? Yes, it is. We know that because we all know relationships where this happens. I have noticed over the years that it seems to happen most often when the couple don't have children. Is this a terrible indictment on having a family? No. What happens, I believe, with couples that don't have children is that they remain more interested in their careers and in their own passions.

Often in a couple with children, one partner – or sometimes both partners – chooses to make their children the primary focus. And there is nothing wrong with that of course, unless they lose interest in their own desires and just become servants. They may be so tired doing a job that can often be tedious – 'drive child to school ... do shopping ...

clean house, etc.' that in the evening they resort to watching TV that they're not interested in. They cease to be interested in themselves in a good way. They cease to be excited by the great joy of being alive and become interested only in their children. It's hard to be attracted and excited by someone who is not excited by life.

It doesn't have to be like this of course. It's perfectly possible to have a family and remain passionate about life – as long as you don't become a victim to the role of 'mother' or 'father.' You're not defined by that role – you are yourself and that person is in love with life. That is attractive. Passion for life is attractive – to me anyway.

Then there is physical desire – which is different. To be a person that is desired sexually, I would argue that you have to pay attention to the senses. At the most simple level, it's hard to desire someone who has bad breath or BO. Then, to be a person that your partner would desire maybe requires a level of sexual confidence and is similar to attraction. If a man or a woman knows that they are good at giving and receiving pleasure and are confident of their sexuality, then it makes them desirable does it not?

Desire is then activated in an animal part of our brains just by the sight of the object of our desire – or the sound of his/her voice or the smell of their skin. Because the body has been programmed to associate sexual pleasure with this person. We are really not so unlike Pavlov's dogs salivating at the sound of a bell rather than the appearance of food. So, in my rather hard-earned opinion, the only way that we can understand pleasure and desire is by bypassing all the externals and getting right to hands-on experience of sexuality and, most often, women's sexuality. That's what we are studying here at the OMX conference. That's why we're here.

• • •

I go to another group OM. I have chosen this man because he doesn't feel threatening to me. I don't yet have the courage to let the men choose me. I just feel the energy and this man felt centred and good.

Again it's hard. I'm surrounded by women who appear to be multi-climactic in this non-goal-centred practice. That may not be so but it appears that way and the amount of noise that some of them make does nothing to ease my feelings of inadequacy. One woman actually said, 'Oh my God!' rather loudly.

But I'm making some progress. I'm focusing on my sensation and there's a moment when I feel a strange opening in my chest and, a wonderful warmth in my arms and legs. It's a silky-smooth ride.

He reports feeling a warmth in his chest too and a glowing feeling from his fingers all the way up his arm.

After each OM you and your partner speak a sensation you had, then you simply say, 'Thank you.' And you move on.

• • •

In the evening Nicole is on the main stage. She is supposed to be giving a talk on OM-based sex but she's on such a high that she just answers questions from the audience instead. They've had six group OM sessions here today. I've been to three and to some of the lectures. I'm guessing that some people skipped the lectures if there was a group OM happening. If a woman is multi-climactic and is having two climaxes per OM (although this is not the intention) and she'd been to all six Oms ... then we can only hope that the men did the grounding properly. There is certainly a lot of oxytocin and dopamine in the air. Everyone is happy and high but the drugs are all internally produced. There isn't a drop of alcohol anywhere.

A woman asks Nicole, 'How can I have sex that is as good as my OM?'

Nicole says, 'You are shifting your centre of gravity with OM to being able to genuinely receive as much pleasure as possible. Often women don't do this in their usual sex lives. Intercourse is a high-level practice but people treat it as if it is a beginner's level practice. So they get beginner's level sex.'

She goes on talking. I give up writing down the questions. I'm making notes for you as fast as I can and writing down anything that may be useful for anyone.

How's this for all of us who are co-dependent?

'Sex with two people trying to get something from each other is like two orphans trying to parent each other.' Ouch.

Or this, even more provocative? 'What we call "love" is often just a contraction. It can be nothing more than a habituated response to the desire for security.' Ouch.

'Monogamy most often doesn't work. Women produce oxytocin at birth and, imagine this, sometimes they have more than one child.' Everyone laughs. Yes, it's true – we can love more than one child but we can only love one man? Marriage, historically, is about the man owning the woman. But now both the man and the woman often feel trapped so how come the status quo allows that?

She says, 'We are the best at what we do here. We have called the conference OM"X" because this is an eXtreme sport. No one is offering you the muzak way of life here.'

I'm scribbling like crazy. My Lamy pen runs out and by the time I've changed my cartridge Nicole is saying,

'The sacred priestesses fucked the war out of the warriors and sent them back into the world as love.'

She tells some great stories about bad sex she's had.

'Men – I would like you to know intuitively that you don't put your dick in my pussy unless my pussy is fully turned on. Slow the shit down.'

The women laugh.

'I've known women who were struggling with mental health issues and they OM for a year and that stuff just burns out – it works its way out of the system.'

That's a pretty amazing claim but we can see that large amounts of sexual pleasure every day in a totally safe environment with no strings attached could make women feel better about a lot of things. Just making the body feel that good every day ... well, I've always said that body, mind and spirit influence each other. I've mainly been speaking about the body point of view about good health and good nutrition but if you add flooding the body twice a day with oxytocin and dopamine that is a real level of happiness in the body. How long could a sad mind continue to feel sad when bathed in pleasure?

I scribble two more notes from Nicole. 'I want my body to be so turned on that I can get off on anyone. I don't want my pleasure to be circumstantial.'

She's certainly radical.

• • •

Naomi Wolf is the final speaker of the evening. Naomi is known for being a courageous feminist whose best-known book *The Beauty Myth* rocketed her to fame when it was first published in 1991. Her most recent book, *Vagina*, which I mentioned earlier, was challenging, hugely important and showed enormous courage so I feel strangely protective of this gutsy New York feminist who needs no protection from me. Tonight, before this audience, she looks happy. No one is going to attack her here. They are just going to listen for anything valuable that she has to say.

Naomi's talk took the audience in directions no other speakers had taken this conference. One of her most scary themes is about the addictive nature of Internet porn and I know that her message hit home.

I know this because 'OneTaste' has its own social media and I read some of the posts from men who had heard what she had said and decided to go cold turkey and stop all Internet porn after the conference. Most movingly one mother wrote that, following Naomi's talk, she had gone home and spoken to her 17-year-old son about porn on the Internet. She had assumed that he would be unable to access it without paying. She had assumed wrong. Following her questions he had broken down and told her everything – how he had started watching it at 12 and become more and more addicted over the years. How he had needed and wanted stronger and stronger images to achieve the same thrills and how now – at 17 – he could no longer get an erection. How he was frightened of interaction with real women. Before this conversation this mother had only read about the desensitizing effects of watching porn – now she had to help her son kick the habit and become comfortable with real women. Very scary stuff. So If you have a son – you may want to have this conversation and not assume that, 'my son wouldn't watch stuff like that'. Yes – he would. At a friend's house, if not at yours.

Aside from the timely and apposite reminder, the main theme that Naomi presents both in her book and on stage is that the importance of the brain/vagina connection has been underestimated. She tells us that 'the vagina is the delivery system for the states of mind that we call confidence, liberation, self-realization and even mysticism.'

When Naomi speaks of the 'vagina', she doesn't mean just the vagina but the whole of the woman's genitals. But Naomi isn't here to talk to us about how to achieve pleasure. Her talk takes the audience in directions no other speakers have taken this conference.

One of the main premises of Naomi's book is that the neural pathways of each woman are different. According to doctors that Naomi interviewed, some of us have more nerve endings in the clitoris, others have more in the vagina, the perineum or the anus. If I have understood her correctly, Nicole wouldn't agree. We hear at OneTaste, again and again, that there are over 8,000 nerve endings in the upper left hand quadrant of clitoris. I'm not interested in argument, I'm interested in learning what works. So when Naomi points out that the G-spot is simply the other end of the same neural pathway as the clitoris – I get out my pen to take notes for us. She is answering questions that the Internet didn't answer when Jovanna and I were discussing jade eggs and G-spots.

How about this one from Naomi: 'Ninety per cent of women in lab conditions, with strangers, reach orgasm when both the area known as the G-spot and the clitoris are stimulated at the same time.' In lab conditions? With strangers? 90%?

It made me smile to think of the men in this audience, thinking, 'Hmmm I wonder what sort of "stimulation" she means.' Many of these men can find an elusive clitoris in the time it would take you and I to find a man's penis. And then they would know how best to stroke it to the width of a millimetre. Naomi is fond of saying that 'our model of female sexuality is 40 years out of date' but this audience is an exception.

One of the other things that Naomi talks about is 'activation'. This is what a woman needs in order to get turned on and it parallels what OneTaste teaches about the 'vigilance centre' of the brain.

'Stress stamps on the autonomic nervous system,' Naomi says. So if a woman is angry with her man she may simply not be able to get turned on. It's not that she's being grumpy or difficult – she's stressed and if she's stressed her vigilance centre can't go down and then it's harder for her to get turned on. I hope you're paying attention here.

Now those of you who are alert will be thinking 'if a woman needs to be so relaxed then where do some women's controversially reported fantasies about rough sex come into this?' And the answer is that a woman can think whatever she likes in the safety of her own bedroom because she knows that she is actually totally safe. It's a fantasy in which she is in total control of the situation. It doesn't mean that she wants to be handled aggressively. That's where the misunderstanding comes in.

The same applies to all the BDSM stuff. Let's go back to Christian Grey in *Fifty Shades* for a second (I confess I only read the first volume) – Christian makes it perfectly clear that Anastasia can leave at any time she wants. They have a code word and any time she says it the whole game is over. So she may be excited – but she is not stressed. It's not the same. She is totally looked after – zero stress.

Looking after your woman and bringing down her stress levels by not being annoying is an important part of activation, Naomi tells us. So men, please, if you want a sexually happy woman in your life, do everything you can to not annoy or stress her. It doesn't serve you.

In an OM, the stroker is trained to say, 'I'm going to touch you now,' before he presses down on her legs to establish the energetic connection. It's all been carefully thought through so that the woman isn't startled even a little bit. And before that – it's the man's job to build the 'nest' – to find the cushions and to make everything perfect for her.

If Naomi had studied OM she would recognize all this as necessary for the kind of 'activation' that has to happen before you even start to ignite a woman's arousal. This is important and, from the point of view of this book, one of the most important things that she speaks about. What do you want to do so that your partner wants to make love to you in the first place? That's back to the subject of desire. The threads are starting to weave together a bit.

The greatest joy for me in watching Naomi is in seeing how much she can let her own guard down in front of this wonderful sexy San Francisco audience. She is now sporting a red armband. Which means, in terms of the conference, that she has been trained to OM. Good for Naomi for having the guts to move beyond the theory. Somehow this place is making everyone very positive and very happy.

At one point Naomi loses her place in her notes and says, 'I've lost my place but I'm doing OK.'

And someone shouts out, 'Yes, you are!' and everyone cheers. This happy audience loves her for her courage. They love her for having the guts to stand on stage in front of this huge audience and talk about sexuality and pleasure.

I had no means of knowing what they had arranged for her or whether they had arranged for one of the more experienced strokers to let her know what all the fuss was about. But she's now wearing an armband and she sure looks happy.

• • •

On Sunday morning I arrive and people are chatting happily, drinking coffee, flirting, wearing, 'Ask me to OM' badges. Just when I was feeling happy Nicole spots me,

'Hi! So awesome to see you here! How are you doing?'

'I, er, I'm finding it quite hard Nicole.'

'You should get your pussy stroked more Isabel. I'll arrange a private OM for you.' (Oh please floor, swallow me up.)

There's a rather good-looking man standing there. She speaks to him – he looks at me, we look at each other. 'Well,' I blush slightly. 'I guess we've been set up.'

'Would you like to OM?' he smiles, sticking to the required request so I'm not obliged to accept.'

'Er ...' (Experience sensation of clenched diaphragm).

Oh, my God. I still have fear in me when I do this with T let alone with a recommended stranger.

'Meet me here just before 11 then?' he smiles flirtatiously.

(Inhalation of breath.) 'Yes, please.' (Notice the heat in the body and a slight nauseous sensation that is usually linked in the body to a fight or flight response.) Then I run away. But only as far as the reception.

I run slap into the people coming out of the group OM. I see one woman coming out on a wheeled walking frame and smile at her. What courage.

'How was it for you?' I ask.

She glances at my name badge. 'Isabel, I am over 70 years old. I graduated from the Institute of Advanced Study of Human Sexuality in 1989, I have serious back problems and I don't care.'

'Really?'

'I never thought I was going to have these new experiences at this age. It was amazing. But please excuse me – I want to attend this next lecture.' And off she wheeled herself.

• • •

It's 10.45am. I'm going to find this stranger in 15 minutes. I have to remember, 'Relax, Open, Breathe.' That's ALL I have to remember. How hard can it be? Why am I afraid? I spot a member of the OneTaste staff, 'What am I afraid of?' 'Desire,' says one. 'Change,' says another. I don't think I'm afraid of either of those. But I have no idea what else it could be. This takes the phrase, 'feel the fear and do it anyway' to a level that I never understood before. Here they want you to focus on the sensation fear produces – just to focus on sensation.

I look into the man's dark brown eyes, 'I'm not bringing any expectations or putting more pressure on myself because Nicole set this up.' Am I trying to convince him or myself?

'I'm just going to OM. It's a goal-less practice.'

'I'm so far outside my comfort zone I feel as if I'm holding on with my toes.'

'What are you holding on for?' He smiles.

'I've no idea.'

So I lie down. And think about surrender. Then I stop thinking. It feels like honey.

• • •

The OM feels expansive. I forget how subtle this is. Maybe fear is of my own expectation. He doesn't rush. He doesn't push. He has no anxiety. He isn't trying to create a good experience for me. He really does 'stroke for his own pleasure' – as the men are taught – but not in any inappropriate 'getting off on it' kind of way – more in a spirit of exploration and connection. At one point he stops stroking completely and I want to laugh because he creates expectation with stillness.

The less he does the more he plays with desire. But he creates the connection first. He puts his finger right on the most sensitive spot and then strokes slowly and softly. This man gives good OM. Quite simply – he knows what he's doing.

I become aware of tension in my neck. I know it's always there, but there is warmth and then suddenly during the OM it starts to hurt like hell.

Yesterday, tears. Another day, awareness that I'm not good at giving adjustments. Another day, warmth and pain. So everything comes up, the mental blocks, the emotional blocks, the physical blocks ... all this you can learn ... through pleasure. How extraordinary is that?

I feel I could live happily in a New York loft with this man for a month and explore the whole OM experience. It's the first OM I've had since being here where I've felt that I could easily do this with him, another hundred times.

I realize now how easy it is for the ego to get in the way of the experience. For the men – they want the woman to have a 'good OM' (in a goal-less practice) partly so that they can feel good about themselves. There is nothing wrong with a man wanting to please a woman or be confident that he is able to do so – but it felt as if this man was beyond all that – he didn't bring his ego into the OM, he just became present. And it's easier to be in an OM that just floats in time and space. I will never see this man again, so I guess it's easier just to float and focus on sensation. I didn't have to think about giving him adjustments, as I'm not training him to please me. I just lay back and enjoyed the ride.

Living in a San Francisco Clitoris
Stroking Community

So it's Monday. The OMX conference is over and I'm settling in to the peace and quiet of living at 1080. I'm glad it's over. All the noise and hype of the conference is far away from the simple and subtle pleasure of the practice. But I missed a few good things yesterday. A lecture from Dr Sara Gottfried on hormone balance and how it affects health and sexuality. The message, as relayed to me second hand, is that stress is bad and raising your oxytocin levels in a safe way is good. Here OMing is the answer to everything. Stressed? OM more. Unhappy? OM more. Sick? OM more. Well, it's free and pleasure feels very good for the body so there is a certain logic to it. I'll read about how to keep my hormone levels healthy later in her book, *The Hormone Cure*.

As I write this, a man walks into the room that I'm actually attracted to. I fix up an OM with him later in the week.

'Would you like to OM?' I ask him. Yayyyy – did it.

'Yes, I would.'

I feel a little warm flush go through me now every time I see him walk past. And this morning one of the other men that live in the San Francisco house that I have a good connection with kissed me on the cheek and I felt a warm sensation pass through my calf muscles. I guess I'm finally tuning in – noticing the sensations in my body, and that I'm alive.

Being in this house is extraordinary.

Let's consider this for a second. The differences between an OM and regular sex are: OM is chosen by both parties on every occasion, a forced OM would be impossible; both parties are always sober (no one drinks before OMing as it's about increased not decreased focus and awareness); the practice takes 15 minutes only so no one feels obliged to buy dinner; the oxytocin is raised easily in women – unlike sex it would be almost impossible for a woman to feel no pleasure during an OM and, if there is climax her dopamine level is raised too; the man knows he is learning as he is watching her vulva for feedback; no one gets pregnant – you don't need to go on the pill, put coils in your body or use condoms; no one has to get jealous as anyone can OM with anyone any time; and the men are needed by the women and appreciated by them. Not too bad huh?

Now before you decide that it really is a cult and I've been totally brainwashed – I am not saying that living in a polyamorous community centred on this practice is any way better than the nuclear family model ... but I am saying that it's certainly not necessarily any worse either.

And is this a cult? Well, it certainly has aspects that feel cult-like but no, it's not a cult, it's a business. For some, it's an alternative lifestyle but for many it's 'only' a sexual practice that teaches women to feel more sexual pleasure and men to feel pleasure through connection.

Why Would You be Afraid of Pleasure?

If I could lead you to a place where, in total safety, you could lie down and have a man who had 20 years of experience in bringing out female pleasure stroke your clitoris for 15 minutes – would you follow me? Would you say, 'Lead the way, Isabel'? Would you say, 'No way. Get away from me with your crazy offers of pleasure'? If the first one is closer to your answer, I'm putting further details in the back of the book. If the second answer is closer to the answer you'd give, then do you know why?

If you are hiding behind 'My partner wouldn't like it.' Well, suppose, just for a moment they supported you unreservedly in doing whatever you needed to do to learn about your own pleasure ... no external impediments ... would you then say – 'OK Isabel, what's the route?'

Or would you stand, like me, rooted to the spot in fear thinking, 'What am I afraid of?'

Am I afraid that the sensation will be too good? Am I afraid of surrender consciously or unconsciously? If we have unconscious fear of surrender, how are we supposed to become conscious of it? Ha ha.

Justine has arranged for me to OM with Ken – the man

they call 'The Master Stroker'. He is the most-experienced man and the top trainer. Of course I'm terrified.

'Why would a woman be afraid of pleasure?' I ask a woman as she walks past me in the OM house.

'Fear of being out of control,' she says, without a moment's hesitation. Hmm, that's the same as surrender again, I guess.

If you're afraid to try any of this – why are you afraid?

I'm still thinking about all this when The Master Stroker himself arrives. He is very short, quiet and full of gentle humility.

'So?' he asks.

I take a deep breath.

'I would love to OM with you, Ken,' I say nervously.

We sit and chat and he tells me that he used to be in computers and had no idea how to connect with women.

'When I learnt this practice,' he says, 'I knew I wanted to make this my life's work.'

So that's what he does. He teaches men how to give women pleasure and he teaches women how to teach the men. I followed him nervously across the building but I'd have followed him nervously across San Francisco or across America if it had been necessary.

• • •

He leads me to a spacious bedroom where a 'nest' is already laid out on the floor. I lie down and he puts on the famous gloves that are so fine that you don't feel them and then applies a little lube to his stroking finger. He puts his finger at the base of my introitus and moves it up slowly till he touches the exact spot on my clitoris that I have been learning is the most sensitive. So easy.

Then, with absolute grace and ease, he simply asks questions. And he asks them in a way that makes it easy for me to answer. He is genuinely demonstrating a goal-less practice – he's just exploring, in the subtlest detail, what pleases me – and so teaching himself.

'Does this feel like a good spot to you?'

'Yes.'

'Does this stroke feel good?'

'Yes.'

'Would you like me to try a little firmer stroke?'

'Yes.'

'Would you like me to back off a little now?'

'No.'

'Would you like a firmer stroke?'

'Yes.'

All the time he's connecting with my energy. He's feeling his way. Suddenly a flash of deep heat starts to rise up through the core of my body. It feels like someone switching on a gas heater that ignites to very hot in just a second.

'And I felt that in my body,' he says gently at the exact moment after my body had gone up 50 degrees. Wow. So this is the 'limbic connection' they talk about. I hadn't moved or made a sound. He really can feel what I'm feeling. Meanwhile he's talking perfectly calmly – just as a masseur might while exploring your shoulders.

'This is a more unusual stroke that is working for you.

It's not one we teach at beginner's level because it would be bad if done clumsily.'

My understanding is that more women, when being stroked, prefer a lighter stroke. A firmer stroke only works if the energetic connection, which can be quite hard to sense, is ignited. If it is not established and the man is not feeling the woman, then a firmer or faster stroke can be frustrating or uncomfortable. Many women know this as they have experienced low or zero sensation from penis thrusting.

But I feel like a radiator on maximum heat and a deep earthy pleasure is still rising.

'Would you like me to back off now?'

'No.'

Sheesh. I'm not feeling any lack of sensation.

'You certainly have sensation.' He smiles.

'Yes.'

'And juice. Everything is working.'

I'm pleased to hear that my body's responding correctly to instructions from my unconscious about which I know nothing.

I feel amazing. And not the least compulsion to push for climax. I feel no need to reach for anything. The whole centre of my body feels as if someone had turned the heat and the bliss level up to about 90%. There's nothing I want or need.

Then the timer goes to tell us that two minutes remain.

'Now I'm going to bring you down with a different stroke.' I've no idea what he's doing but it feels a bit like being lowered gently and placed on a descending cloud. We finish the OM formally. The practice requires that I say, 'There was a moment when ...' and describe a sensation. I say, 'There was a moment when the whole inner core of my body heated up.'

He says, 'There was a moment when your clitoris got longer and firmer and I could tell at the point of contact that we were going in the right direction. But then I started to feel a warm velvety glow in the small of my back and I knew that we had entered a state of ignition.'

I feel a little woozy.

'That was so simple. You just established a clear connection and then asked questions that it was easy for me to answer. You made it so easy. I've been having such trouble trying to feel the sensations clearly enough to give the adjustments. My strokers haven't had a clear sense of what kind of stroke to give and I haven't had a clear sense of how to guide them. It's been like the blind leading the blind. But with you it was all suddenly beautifully easy.'

'Let me stop you there.' He smiles. 'There are two dangers with you OMing with someone they call "The Master Stroker". The first is that you make it about me and the second is that you try to re-create the experience. Now that you've felt what is possible it means that you have a responsibility to teach men how to do that for you.'

'I know. It seems I'm a poor teacher.'

'Also don't try and re-create that OM because every OM is different.'

'Yes,' I sigh. 'Most of them, in my case, with a lot less sensation.'

'Just try giving a wider range of adjustments. Tell your

OMing partners, "I'm working on giving more adjustments," and then try, "Could you try a firmer stroke?" Or, "Could you try a lighter stroke?" Or, "Could you try a faster or slower stroke?"'

All this time, I realize, and despite all this training, I have been making the same mistake so many women make of hoping the man will know what to do by some kind of intuition.

And even Ken. He hadn't put his finger down and known what to do by magic or intuition – he had simply asked questions in a way that had made it easy for me to answer them. The master as a beginner... 'Zen mind – beginner's mind.' Clear – without ego and trained. What a joy.

I am so glad to be in the present. I thank Ken for the OM and leave remembering that I had been fearful all day before an OM in which I'd had deeper sensation than ever before. I felt a hot sensation deep inside me for about an hour after this OM. He hadn't touched me internally at all but it felt, as they say here, 'like, totally awesome.'

And still I'm not sure why or what I'm learning. What had he said? 'Now it's just about training every other stroker'. So I can't OM with Ken every day for the rest of my time in San Francisco? Damn.

• • •

Tonight, one of the other girls from London arrives in my room. The house is very full and Emma, who is one of the youngest of us and is learning all this at 24, had been sleeping on a floor somewhere. We compare experiences.

'I had the most terrible OM yesterday.' She laughs. 'It was some guy who was new. I don't know why I said, "Yes."'

I laugh. I'm dreading what she's going to say next.

'He was actually stroking my outer labia. I mean, they did have diagrams up at the conference that showed clearly where the clitoris is. I just gave up. He was a lost cause.'

'You're so funny. That's cruel. After all, the poor bloke was at least there to learn.'

'Yes, but I'd had a hard day. If he hadn't even worked out that the point he was supposed to be aiming at is at least somewhere central, it wasn't my problem.'

I'm afraid we both laughed.

'I decided it was the next girl's problem. I mean, the women here have more patience than I do.'

'So you just lay there for the entire 15 minutes?'

'Yes. A kind of existential despair set in. I came to a greater and greater realization that he really was that far off. Maybe he fell asleep on the training day?'

'Oh dear.'

'And there was another man who I said "Yes" to who was about 60 and he was so fumbly. I wondered what he'd been doing all his life. I thought he'd have some experience but he had no idea how to please a woman.'

'There are millions of men out there with no idea how to please a woman, Emma.'

'And there was this one man... I'm sure he fell asleep.'

I laughed. 'Yes, there's a man in London who I think dozed off in an OM with me once. It's not very flattering is it? I mean this is my clitoris after all. It's been quite a journey to get myself to the place where I'm able to do this. You'd think the least he could do would be to stay awake. I mean, dozing off during a cross-legged meditation on the breath is one thing. But dozing off while he's supposed to be focused on my clitoris is another.'

'Quite.'

'I know I shouldn't ask but ... who was it?' We started to laugh rather hysterically. And inevitably discovered it was the same stroker. Not many men take a doze during an OM.

Emma suddenly said, 'Oh my God, I could never tell my mother these things.'

My worry was a little different, 'I could never tell my daughter these things.'

'My mother would never believe this. She'd be horrified.'

'My daughter would never believe this. She'd be horrified.'

• • •

My time at the 1080 OM house is drawing to a close. So, what have I learnt? I'm trying to draw it all together. For me and, hopefully, you too. The message – 'You are 100% responsible for what happens in your life' – may seem like an annoying and banal platitude from the American positive thinking movement. It certainly seemed that way to me. I remember how I battled against it when I first heard it. Gradually I understood. We are not 100% responsible for what happens. But we are obviously 100% responsible for how we respond to what happens. The more I took responsibility for my life and the more I saw myself as the creator of it the better I felt and the better my life became. Very annoying.

But I didn't apply this to sexuality. Because it takes two, I went on thinking that I needed the right man to come along before I could sort all this out. What was I waiting for? A man who I imagined would be an intuitive of some kind? Who would understand my body even though I didn't understand it myself?

'Ah well, hello Mr Christian.' – *Fifty Shades of Grey* – 'I'm a virgin you see.' The stuff of fiction?

This is one area where, while, in theory I'm aiming at 100% responsibility, I still somehow find myself imagining there is a man who knows what to do in an OM or in bed without me having to communicate clearly to him. I know some of my readers are laughing at me, 'but Isabel, we knew this years ago.' Most men and some women discover their pleasure and how to maintain it at a young age. Yes, my happy brothers and sexually turned on and happy sisters – you are out there – good for you. And if you are married and in this happy situation then I celebrate for you and hope that you successfully maintain your pleasure.

For the rest of us it still seems that many women are settling for second-rate sex. Women have to stop putting men's pleasure before their own.

If we want to turn around the statistic that 60% would rather be cuddled than have sex, we have to do something different. It's too easy to blame men for being clumsy, selfish or incompetent. We have to take 100% responsibility for our experience in life, in a bed or in an OM nest. Or at least I do.

• • •

There's a man sitting in the common room sobbing. Someone told me that he is breaking his heart over a relationship. I know what that feels like. There is no chance to indulge in the illusion of ownership here. But I remember the sensation of a broken heart. An ache between the breastbones and feeling that life is unbearable if you can't be with just that one person. You know that sensation, right? I remember how painful it is. When it goes quiet I speak to him.

'Would you like to OM? I need a number one for morning practice tomorrow.'

'OK,' he says, and makes a note on his phone with marginally less enthusiasm than you'd make an appointment with your taxman.

OK, he's busy with his broken heart and the guys that live at 1080 do this a lot. But all the same – I think it's fair to expect just a glimmer of something if I've invited a man to stroke my clitoris. If he doesn't feel like it that's OK too. Hmmm. How to re-negotiate?

An hour later I look for him and find him. 'About our OM ...' I speak up rather bravely, 'I've changed my mind.' He just looks at me. 'OK, then. As you wish.' He doesn't ask for an explanation. I launch into one anyway.

'It's just that, when I asked, you seemed so disinterested ... I wondered whether you really want to ... or whether you just said "yes" because you need two partners for the practice?'

Silence.

'I mean this may happen every day for you, but for me

this is still a big deal and if you don't want to OM with me ...'

'Stop. I do. I do want to OM with you.'

'I didn't think it was personal. I didn't think it was about me. I wasn't sure, from your response, that you want to OM at all.'

'Yes. I do. I do want to OM. And I'd like to OM with you. Please. I'm just not myself this week. There was a woman you see ...' his voice peters out.

'Oh, yes. There was a woman ... She's just another woman, you know. There are lots of us. (I talk as if I've not broken my heart over a man.) We are each special in our own way.'

'Yes. And I'd like to OM with you.'

That's all I want. To know that he really is a 'yes'.

'OK, then. As you ask so nicely.'

• • •

He's my number one at the practice this morning. I lie down and he does all the usual prep. He slides his finger with the lube on from the bottom to the top of my introitus and finds the most sensitive spot with a mixture of good training and the light in the room that means he can see.

Then he starts to play me. This rather broken-hearted man starts to play and somehow hits 'ignite'. As he strokes I can feel my body start to heat up and that this pleasure is somehow shared by him. Then there is a loop; I get more aroused because he's aroused, because I'm aroused. Mmmmm. His focus is 100% and he just seems to know how to play. He has what they call an 'upstroke' that takes me effortlessly upwards, a feeling of going up and still further up as the sensation becomes more and more intense – hotter and closer somehow, a focused sensation in my clitoris but one that creates heat through my body until I tingle and every part of every limb feels as though it's singing.

Then just at the point where he seems to reach the very peak of possible sensation – he changes to a downstroke – like a rollercoaster, down I come. I breathe out heavily and groan as I come down, the heat drains away and instead there's a kind of grounded earthy feeling. I'm holding onto his leg as if it's the safety bar on the rollercoaster.

He changes the stroke again – heaven knows what he's doing.

'I'm supposed to be practising giving adjustments,' I gasp.

'I don't want to discourage you from verbal adjustments,' he says, 'but I'm watching your pussy,' and takes me up again. Somehow the electricity from my clitoris fires up my body with buzzy heat. Then, effortlessly, he seemed to go on with some kind of upstroke. By this time, I'm unaware of the room or anyone else there or asking for anything – I just want him to keep doing what he's doing.

He's breathing heavily himself and rather satisfying sounds are coming out of him. I give up holding on even with my toes. Sure enough he's able to keep on with his upstroke and keep on with his upstroke and keep on with his upstroke. Until there – as a treat in this goal-less practice – he obviously decides to do what they call here 'take me over.' I kick and groan as my body convulses with heat and electricity. I'm amazed that my body can produce such a simple and sassy climax in about eight minutes. I'm afraid I may have made a little bit of noise. I hope I haven't disturbed any of the other strokers or strokees.

And even then my 15 minutes isn't up. He switches to downstrokes and brings me flying down until he has gentle groans coming out of me from somewhere. Then he just takes me on a little glider ride for the remainder of the time. I sit up at the end. 'Er – there was a moment when ...' I laugh, as I don't have a sensation to describe. I can't think of anything to say but my face is very red. He tells me his sensation, but my ears aren't working.

'You need to learn to breathe more fully and never hold your breath. It will increase your sensation considerably.'

'Er – yes. Thank you. Er – what was your name again?'

He smiles. 'It's not about me.'

Back in my room I email Ken and tell him about this resonant OM.

'I thought I was learning about giving adjustments? I didn't give him any. So what am I supposed to be learning now?'

'To enjoy.'

Ah, yes. To enjoy. Pleasure. That's what we're studying, isn't it?

Unsurprisingly – if you can find a way to explore this, I recommend this practice.

Autumn in Shades of Red

Yoni Healing Anyone?

It's autumn and I'm turning my attention to an even more difficult subject than the external part of the clitoris: the part of my body that contains the greater area of the clitoris – the vagina. Did you also know that there are heterosexual women all over Europe that meet together to massage inside each other? I am not making this up – this could be happening in a town near you. And more than this – that there is Yoni worship going on? I thought that some of the events I've been exploring this year were quite unusual. But you never know what people are getting up to.

I had to go to the dentist for a check-up today. This is the third time I have met this new woman dentist.

I arrived. They are always friendly. 'Good morning Isabel. How are you? You're looking well.'

'Good morning, Katherine. Thank you. Yes, I'm good. You're looking amazing, as usual. I always have the impression that you glow somehow. Is dentistry, the way you do it, a particularly relaxing job?'

'As you ask ...' she says, showing me to my chair and pressing a button to make me horizontal, 'I've just had a mouth massage.'

'A what?'

'It's a massage on the inside of the mouth. Put these

glasses on please. It's very relaxing having the inside of the mouth massaged. Strangely so. It's not something I'd had before. The inside of the mouth is very sensitive.'

'Ah, but have you had your yoni massaged?' I asked, attracting a surprised reaction from the dental nurse.

I suppose I expected her to say 'What's a yoni?' as most people don't even know the word. I explain that although 'phallic' meaning 'in the shape of a phallus' is a word we all know, 'yonic' meaning 'in the shape of yoni' isn't a word many people know. But she was way ahead of me. She said,

'Oh yes, and worshipped too. And open your mouth wide please.'

'Waaaat?' I tried to say while she peered attentively into my mouth.

'My yoni has been not only massaged, but worshipped. On an altar, with rose petals. ... Upper left 8 watch occlusal,' She instructed her dental nurse.

'Ahhhhhh?'

'And with women chanting, praying and meditating ... Upper 7 OK. Upper 6 OK ... And then they came forward and knelt down in front of my yoni while I was lying naked on a stage with my legs apart ... Upper left 5 porcelain crown.'

'Oan a haaaage?'

'Yes, on a stage. The women come forward and offer rose petals ... Upper left 3 to upper right 3, OK ... To be fair I was one of five women on the stage having their yonis worshipped.'

You probably think I'm making this up, don't you? But no! My dentist has had her yoni worshipped.

'Upper right 4 watch occlusal.'

'Oere oas 'is?' I asked.

'The place was perfect actually. It was at the Inns of Court with all the old judges staring down at us from the walls ... 5 –7 OK. Upper right 8 missing.'

She took a brief break, allowing me to speak.

'I don't understand. How have I not heard about this? I mean has everyone heard about this? Have you had your yoni worshipped too?' I turned to the dental nurse who just giggled behind her face-mask. 'I'll take that as a "yes" then? Who hires out the Inns of Court for yoni worship?'

'And open please. It's part of the London Tantra Festival. It happens every year. Surely you must have been? ... Lower left 7 needs composite filling.'

'Oww hid uuu heeeee ahou 'is?' I asked.

'Watch lower left 6. Lower left 5 to lower right 5 OK ... I hooked up with this random guy for a one-night stand and he was a tantric practitioner ... Do you floss daily? You must floss daily ... He was inside me with an erection for four or five hours after spending about 2 hours preparing me. I had about six orgasms. It was the most remarkable night of my life. So that interested me in tantra ... Lower right 6 watch occlusal.'

'Yeh – I han hee aaa aaa ould oo iat.'

'You'll have to make an appointment for a filling.' She pressed a button restoring me to a sitting position.

'Did you take his number?'

'We could have had a relationship but I said "no" – the sex was amazing but he wasn't right for me. But that's what interested me in tantra, which led to the yoni worship.'

'Really great to see you, Isabel.'

'Hello, how are you?' She said turning to her next patient. I wonder does she has conversations like this with all her patients? I had to go and have a coffee to recover from this conversation. I emailed her and asked her if I could include this story in a book I was writing. And whether I could use her real name. 'Oh yes, that's fine.' So there it is. You can look up Tantra Festivals near you if you don't believe me.

But where was I? Ah yes, the yoni. As a person familiar with various kinds of spiritual and 'New Age' thought (I am making this assumption about you – forgive me) you may be familiar with the idea that the body holds memories as well as the brain. You may even have heard the theory that cells store memories. I don't mean genetic information, I mean a kind of 'memory' of trauma. This is known as pseudoscience; although many people believe it there is no known way of measuring whether this is so or not. The evidence is anecdotal. The problem with anecdotal evidence is that there are sometimes thousands of people who share the same beliefs and the same experiences. So what is 'true' and what is not? This is the current situation with what they call 'yoni massage'.

I am told (and I have no reason to believe or disbelieve) that the walls of the vagina store trauma. So, just as people who feel, or have felt, they have the world on their shoulders often become stooped ... so those that have had bad sexual experiences can later experience pain or numbness instead of pleasure when the inside of the vagina is touched, even with a loving and sensitive partner. Assuming that she may have had therapy and done the work needed to bring her consciousness in line with her present circumstances as well as she can – we are told that memory is still stored in the vaginal walls. Furthermore, we're assured that a form of pressure massage can release these memories. Which is why there are women massaging each other internally. They claim this yoni massage is a source not only of pleasure but also of healing.

I bet some of you think I'm making this up. But in Germany, I am reliably informed, 'all the women seem to be working on each other'. But that may be a slight exaggeration.

I have to confess that I experienced this – such is my commitment to experiential research but it did not provide any healing nor memories that I cherish.

A while later I attended a workshop with a group of women and we were paired at random by drawing names out of a hat. The process was called 'yoni healing'. Immediately my hackles were raised. 'Yoni massage' would have been less irritating to me, but to claim that this process is a form of healing ... well, as far as I'm concerned, the jury is still out. You could give me a great shoulder massage or an all-over body massage and I'm going to enjoy it very much. But even the most experienced body masseur isn't going to call it a 'body healing'. Why, just because it's the yoni being massaged, has it become 'healing'?

As some of you will observe, these thoughts will not have put me in a very receptive mood for the experience. I had been partnered, by the random draw, with a woman who was in her 60s and it was her first ever experience either of being touched or of touching another woman in this way. I suppose neither of us were ideal students. We followed the instructions – massaging first the stomach then the muscles at the top of the legs, the inside of the legs, the outer labia, the inner labia and finally internally.

Various women in the room at the time had different experiences. Some cried, some shouted out in pain, some gave groans of pleasure. Those massaging were very caring – it was impossible not to notice that. And what did I experience? Well, I'm pretty sure I can sum it up without too much fear of exaggeration – nothing. And what did she experience when I was massaging her? Nothing. And why would this have been so? I think it's because my main intention was not to 'release trauma'. I have no belief that I'm able to do that, but my aim was simply to make sure that her experience was gentle and not to hurt her. She similarly was very gentle and obviously didn't want to hurt me.

I don't want to put you off doing workshops in Europe, the US or Asia. There are many kinds of workshops that explore sexuality where this will not be on the agenda. But if you study sexuality with a group of women to a reasonably high level you are expected to leave your inhibitions behind and get in touch with your body– so sooner or later this will show up as it is considered, by many, to be a necessary part of women's sexual healing. The presumption is that women are in need of healing. I have never heard of any woman being told, 'Oh, you don't need this. You're fine.' To be fair though, some women I've spoken to that have done different kinds of workshops in various countries have had experiences that they describe as 'transformative'.

'It depends who does it,' says one of my German friends on the telephone. 'I've done this five times. With an osteopath, my experience was that the first time my cervix felt fixed and he seemed to be able to make it less rigid. The second time he released tension, and the third time he did a kind of trauma work and that seemed to release something too. But I've also done this with less experienced people and it's done nothing.'

'And were these treatments from men or women?'

'I've had yoni massage from men and women. That doesn't really matter. It's the experience of the practitioner that counts.'

With some women – in Germany, the UK and the US – this is so popular that there are regular groups where women meet for yoni massage. If you are a man reading this – before you ask – no, men are not allowed to go and watch.

I went up to the person running the workshop and asked, 'So – everyone else seemed to be having a far more profound experience than I had. Does that mean that I'm less fucked up than the other women as I certainly felt no need to cry, sob, shout out, swear or any of the other reactions that we saw? Or does it mean that I'm more fucked up?'

'Oh, you are more armoured.' I was told. That's 'New Age' speak for more fucked up. Well, to be a little more specific – the idea is one that originally came from Wilhelm Reich, who died in 1957, that as bad things happen to you physically you form body armour. So you are less able to feel. It makes a certain amount of sense. My problems with this theory are: firstly, why is it that some people who have had the most reasons to create heavy armour, for example those who may have suffered sexual abuse, will still have sensitivity? Women who have been in bad, loveless marriages for years can re-marry and discover a whole new experience of pleasure that they didn't know was possible for them. I know some women who admit to being very messed up emotionally and yet they have very good sex lives. Surely if this tendency to 'armour' the inside of our vaginas was universal it would be more widely known? Women would be talking about it at the pub, 'I have this terrible knot in my fanny armour.' And if releasing inner knots were a simple path to better orgasms – then surely more people would be making money providing this service and it would be written about on the cover of *Cosmopolitan* with predictable regularity?

But – to be fair, I must put my scepticism aside, realizing that I know nothing about this subject. To be as open as possible – if this yoni healing had been offered to me by someone who had trained for many years, and had massaged as many yonis as Nicole has stroked clitorises (I so wish that the plural was clitori), then I would be listening more carefully. But, should I believe a diagnosis from a woman running a workshop who was at the other end of the room at the time and is basing her statement on the fact that I had very little feeling when a totally untrained woman was touching me very gently trying not to hurt me? I'll pass.

I am not in the business of going to workshops to collect new limiting beliefs. When I got back from the workshop

I rang my old friend William Bloom (author of about a million books on all things alternative – founder in the 1980s of 'Alternatives' in London and general knower of all things) and he said, 'You should sue them.' He didn't mean it, as everyone in the alternative world is aware that what we do and what we believe is our responsibility – but he made me feel better.

Because of course I did wonder whether she's right. Maybe this is the reason why I'm one of the many women who doesn't experience orgasm during penetration. Maybe I'm more than averagely numb? Another sign, apparently, that I'm messed up is that I don't want my yoni massaged by a woman anyway. According to the women I've met who practise this – most women feel safer when they know that their genitals are not being touched with any sexual intent but purely for the purpose of healing.

'But I like men.' I reply pathetically. The women look at me with pity. It's just sensation after all. And I did experience this when, despite not really having any desire to do so, I agreed to have an OM with Rachael. It felt just the same. I didn't like it as much though.

I've just read a book called *Yoni Massage: Awakening Female Sexual Energy*. Unsurprisingly, it's translated from the German. I'm not sure how many books on yoni healing you could sell in the UK. I don't think many mainstream publishers would be competing. The author, Michaela Riedl[15], runs one-to-one sessions where women go to her and, for between three and three-and-a-half hours, receive massage first of themselves, then of their external genitals, then internally. Michaela is straight and so are the women that go to her. Am I more than usually inhibited, do you think? Is this idea of exploring your sexuality and your body sensation away from the presence of men appealing to you? Or not?

If you hate the idea there are some people who might jump to the conclusion that you have issues that you need to overcome. And to be fair you may have. On the other hand, if you are heterosexual and hate the idea of any kind of exploration of your sexuality in a mixed group they may be concerned for you for that reason. The ideal, apparently, is that we become sexually comfortable enough that we are open to either option. After all, we are not talking about having sex here – we are talking about massage of a part of the body for the purpose of understanding and healing.

Women are wonderful, beautiful, sexy, intelligent creatures and they understand how other women's bodies work. I have had some experience of the beauty of women's work in the workshops that I did with Shakti Tantra. There is a feeling of being safe – of vulnerability – a beautiful way of being sexually that maybe can only be found when no one has any sexual needs or expectations of anyone else. So I would say that if the idea of being in a group of women scares you – go immediately and find out why.

But everyone has limits and when I had a woman's fingers up my fanny I felt I'd reached them. And if I'm going to explore this any further – it has to be with an experienced practitioner – so I know I can trust what they say. And, for my preference, male.

• • •

Looking for 'yoni healing', other than through personal recommendation, is not a piece of research for the fainthearted. Before beginning a search, the computer should flag up a liability warning and you should have to declare that you are over 18, and a fully responsible adult. You have to be able to tell the sheep from the goats in a country where they all look very much the same.

Putting 'yoni massage' into Google is likely to draw up a number of sites that look as if they are run by some kind of tantric practitioners. This is where you should take a pinch of salt, become as sceptical as possible and use every ounce of common sense that you have available to you. Ignore anything that says 'free sensual yoni massage for ladies.' Ha ha.

The first site that I find is using lots of words like 'kundalini' and 'yonic', but on a quick browse you soon realize that the main service on offer is visits to a hotel room, the man's face is not pictured, he will light candles to 'warmify' the atmosphere and that a 'wine ritual' is part of the erotic massage. He further promises that 'erotic yoni massage' is a 'spiritual stimulation' and promises that he will 'take you out of this universe with joyful pleasure'. He adds not to ring the number directly but only contact him by text. Ha ha ha.

I searched 'yoni massage Glasgow', 'yoni massage Belfast', 'yoni massage Edinburgh' and finally 'yoni massage London'. It didn't take me long to work out who was offering genuine therapeutic work and who was offering a 'service for the frustrated lady'. This is why I would say, don't start the journey here and don't go to see any alternative sexual health practitioner other than through personal recommendation.

But I am about to break this rule myself. Following a couple of hours on the Internet I finally find a practitioner that I like the sound of. His site contains the question, 'What is tantric massage?' And he replies, 'Many things go under this name these days. Some people offer a full body massage including stroking the genitals, other people present it as chakra balancing, sometimes it's even a euphemism for sex for sale.' He goes on, 'My tantric massage for women is serious and professional expert bodywork which guides you toward expanded, healthy, profound and wholesome sexuality in your daily life.'

His site contains a full head and shoulders picture of him, statements from many women and the offer to speak with any of them on the telephone. I didn't, but the fact that I could have rung him and said, 'I'd like to speak to three women that you have worked with,' is reassuring.[16]

But now – here is the controversial bit where I'm going to make myself unpopular with some people that work in this profession – this man has a whole page on why it makes more sense for a heterosexual woman to go to a heterosexual male practitioner. He writes, to paraphrase, that it's sexual energy that you are learning to understand. He states that many people believe that a man offering this kind of bodywork has his own agenda. But I don't think that's necessarily so. It's not a question of him wanting anything from the women that go to him – and he's very careful to point out that he has a loving partner – but simply that a heterosexual male has a certain energy.

This matches my feelings and experience. I don't feel as comfortable having my vagina touched or massaged by women. His site says,

'I am constantly surprised by heterosexual female practitioners offering this experience to heterosexual women. To me it appears to be a deep misunderstanding of sexuality bodywork. There are many ways sexuality can be addressed – psychology, tantra workshops, counselling, educative media – where a woman helping a woman makes sense in a "me too" way. A sensual massage however is direct experience through the body and out of the mind. Of course if you are gay, you will be energetically comfortable being massaged by a woman.'

Many professional body workers will not agree with this. They teach, 'Learn about your body from another woman and when you are happy and content you can go to a man and gently and confidently teach him how to please you.' Yes, I understand. I get the theory. But it just doesn't feel right for me.

At another women's workshop my greatest fear was realized. It was almost dark and the room was lit only by candles and it was the end of the day ... but as one process led into another I realized, to my horror, that I was going to be expected to masturbate in a room with other people. The fact that they were women didn't make me feel any more comfortable.

This wasn't in California or even New York; this was in

Europe. There was music playing and we were being invited gently to 'explore our pleasure' making active positive use of exhibitionism and voyeurism. We were being encouraged to look at each other. A woman beside me was bravely standing and stroking herself. Well, I say 'bravely' but maybe it wasn't brave for her – maybe she was enjoying the exhibitionism in the entirely positive and natural way that they were encouraging, but I hated it. There was a kind of magnificence about her in the half light, she was completely naked and with her eyes closed she was standing and stroking her breasts and her genitals and I was sitting on the floor wondering whether to look or not to look. I was being encouraged to look but I didn't want to.

She seemed to being enjoying knowing that there may have been 19, 20, 30 pairs of eyes upon her. In a corner another woman was sobbing and not rubbing anything except her eyes. Behind me, another woman, who I knew was gay and so may have been enjoying all this female sexual energy more than I was, was masturbating joyfully and making sounds of rapture. It was all working for her at least.

Meanwhile I was thinking, Am I supposed to be aroused by the energy in the room? I have no idea if I'd have been any happier if there had been men present. This was certainly safe but it just didn't feel right to me.

So anyway – here is a man on a very professional site, with all the references I could ask for, sticking his neck above the water and saying something that, to me, makes complete sense. So I rang him, had a long conversation and found out what he charges for this kind of bodywork. It seemed a reasonable price. I could save up and I could go. If you want to perhaps you could save up and go.

Now I just have to find a way to explain this to T.

T says, 'It was bad enough when you were in San Francisco. What exactly is this bodywork going to involve?'

'I don't know, T. I didn't ask too many specific questions. I was afraid that if I found out too much I'd be too scared to go. Apparently there is a lot of talking and if anything doesn't feel right I can simply walk out of the door.'

'Well, OK. As long as you're totally happy. Just don't let me know when you are going. I won't be able to concentrate on my job. When is it? No, no. I don't want to know. Where is it? ...'

'What difference does it make to you whether it's in Edinburgh or St Ives?'

'None. None. You're right. I don't want to know where it is. When is it again? What does it involve? Can I see his website?'

'You really want to know?'

'No, I don't.'

'He also teaches tantric massage for couples. Are you interested?'

'If I can stop hyperventilating then, yes, I'd love to learn. You want to do this with me?'

'Maybe.'

Tantric Massage and Light Beams

OK. We are back in the present. Don't you find that with life?

I don't know what I'm expecting. It's best to have no expectations. If anything happens that I'm not happy about I'll just say 'enough' or 'thank you – stop'. If I'm unhappy, I'll leave. I can remember that from Sue's workshop. The clear use of the word 'no'.

I'm in a leafy road of huge, elegant houses in North London. Most of these big old houses, like the one that I've arrived at, are now divided into flats. I walk up to the door and a gentle face appears from a room where it seems to be evening – even though it's 11am outside. In a tantric world it's perpetually early dusk – the crepuscule, before it feels late, when there is still plenty of time.

An attractive, round-looking face greets me. He could be anywhere between 30 and 40 – impossible to guess. He looks young but has the centred and grounded energy of an older man. He smiles with a mixture of confidence and shyness.

'My name is Alexey.'

I hold out my hand, friendly Labrador style.

'Hello Alexey, my name's Isabel. This feels very strange. But I suppose everyone says that.'

'Yes. Apparently I'm a very scary person because everyone is terrified before they come. Some people want to run away when they come for the first time.'

'I don't want to run away.' I pause. 'Not yet anyway.'

The room is decorated tastefully with deep colours and gentle music of the subtle 'New-Agey' kind is playing. Not tweety birds like the plinky-plink they play in beauty salons, just relaxing.

'Would you like coffee?'

Someone speaking these words is always a good sign.

'Yes, please.'

And then we sit and talk. We talk for two hours. And I find I agree with 100% of what he says. I wish this were an interview because I want to write everything down. But I'm not going to tell him, initially, that I'm writing. I don't want to make him nervous. So I just listen and he talks complete sense. I can disagree with almost anyone but not today, it seems. I want to curl up on his sofa and sleep. His energy feels cosy, safe and comforting. Either that or his gas fire has burnt all the oxygen in the room. I tell him I felt uncomfortable exploring my sexuality with women.

'You're heterosexual.'

I laughed. 'I know! And my boyfriend says that when he did a weekend of men's work, the closest they got to touching each other was punching each other's hands to help them express anger.'

I think it may be some years until we hear of a workshop of straight men helping each other heal their 'lingams' with touch.

'Sex is about energy,' he says. 'Not just physical release of tension – which is the way that it is so often used today. It's about saturating each other with beautiful energy – all this magnetism, sensation, vibration between your bodies. And the yoni has the most powerful energy. It is designed for that connection and you don't have the same energy in your hands or in your mouth. Love in sex is energy too. You feed each other with the energy of love from your body – and when you give love like this, you do it just as much for yourself as you do for the other person.'

Makes sense to me.

I tell him about my summer. About my experience with the clitoral strokers of San Francisco and he says that the new emancipation of the clitoris is both a good thing and a bad thing. I defend it:

'So many women have no pleasure. At least training men to find the clitoris and to stroke it means that women have pleasure.'

This is true, but it's very similar to the male penis. It is, essentially, a penis. It has the same innervation and the same energy, and when women focus on it they are connecting more with a male energy within them and not their true nature. The yoni is the true female organ and it can offer a richness of female sexual experience – if women develop it but often, instead, they choose a clitoral pleasure. You simply irritate the nerve, it stays irritated until you relieve it.

'Irritate the nerve?' Ha ha ha. That's what we've been learning? How to irritate the nerve effectively?

'Well, that's what people are doing when they rub and rub as if it was only about physical technique. Physiological response is not what human pleasure is about. Sexual energy is vibrations. Sensation is a vibration between the energies of two people. The yoni holds a richness of vibrations. One needs to learn how to create the right energy there.'

'But I've been told that many of our vaginas are damaged.

There is this idea that knots develop in the vaginal walls and need to be released through massage?'

'I have only been doing this work for ten years but I would say that I don't see any proof of that. It's not what I do.'

'So, what do you use?'

'Energy and vibration. Sensation is a form of vibration. A response to the energy of the other person.'

'This makes complete sense and matches my experience.'

I find myself thinking of the saying of Jill Bolte Taylor: 'Please be responsible for the energy you bring into this place.'

'So you would say, "Sex is energy"?'

'Yes, because otherwise all you have is physiology.'

'And how would you define good sex then?'

'Good sex is something that brings beauty, positive energy and love into your life.'

I like this definition because it includes the results of the sex as well as the sex itself.

He asks me about my sex life and I tell him everything I'm experiencing with T. All the complexity you'd expect between two people.

What a weird job he has. He listens and eventually speaks.

'One of the great things about sex is that you can give unconditional love in sex, whereas relationships are complicated. When you give love in sex you do it just as much for yourself as for the other.'

'Presumably though, you need to be reasonably OK in yourself before you can love someone else? Otherwise, as Nicole says, it's like two orphans trying to parent each other?'

'You need to be conscious of what kind of energy you are giving out of your body and know that your partner needs your love. This is the highest nature of a woman – to radiate physical love as sexual energy, as sunshine to her partner. To be a creator, a nurturer, a giver of life. All women have it within and feel grounded and confident when they connect with this energy. Just as he is able to give her love with his body.'

'Hmm. I don't get many letters from women who describe their sex lives like this. What's the main thing that women need to learn?'

'Women are too passive in creating the right kind of sex lives for themselves. They don't take responsibility. The sexual journey is about each individual woman. It's what you're learning.'

'Yes, that's why I'm here.'

'OK, so let's do the massage.'

'This is the point where some women leave, right?' I stand up, breathe deeply and glance at the door. Outside the sun is shining. I do feel like bolting.

'Let me just tell you about what will happen,' he says.

'First of all, you are not here to have an orgasm.' Might as well go then. Not really. I sit down again.

'Experiences like this may occur but it's not about that. So you can put that out of your head.'

'OK.'

'We are exploring vibration and sensation. I'd like you to look for the sensation of happiness not for the sensation of excitement.'

Hmmm ... post-OM training I'm quite experienced in looking at sensation. I don't think happiness is a sensation but I decide not to argue at this point.

'OK.'

'You may experience different kinds of noise in your head. There is what I call irrelevant noise – such as, you may find yourself thinking about things far away from here in the past or the future or in a different geographical location. Or there is noise which you may feel is relevant, for example – "I wonder if my thigh looks weird from that angle?" or "What is he going to do next?" This is all just noise. None of it is relevant. Just focus on sensation.'

'This is the same as in an OM.'

'OK.'

'I'll be talking to you during the massage but you don't need to reply. Obviously if there is anything that you don't like or you're not comfortable with in any way just ask me to stop.'

'Yes.'

'When we come to the yoni part of the massage it's important that you draw the sensation up to the heart.'

'With the breath?'

'Yes. You know the point they call the heart?'

'Yes, it's the spot between your breasts that hurts when someone you love goes away.'

'That's it. Draw the sensation, the energy, up to there. After that it will look after itself.'

'OK.'

He leaves the room and I undress and clamber onto his

massage table to lie face down on the stretchy towelling table cover.

I've had lots of massage. This is different. It's not the sexual massage of those that hold their hands six inches over a woman's body and make some woman orgasm without touch. (Yes, this is possible but that's another story. You can look up The Tantric Mongoose[17] or Sasha Cobra[18] on Google later. I think it's mainly projection.) Nor is it Reiki, where people move their hands in what they call your energy field, nor is it a Kahuna-type massage where all the action seems to be in the masseur.

He comes back, puts one hand on my back and with his other hand holds my hand and talks to me. I don't remember what he says – but his tone of voice is warm and he makes me feel relaxed and calm. Then he puts both hands on my lower back and just holds them there while I feel the warm energy move through me. The massage is slow with no pushing or downward pressure. This isn't a massage to relieve sore muscles. This is a massage to help me tune into subtle sensations. He moves a finger just a little and I feel a warm echo somewhere inside me.

Then I find myself thinking about San Francisco. I wonder how they all are.

'Only the present moment. Nothing else is real,' I hear Alexey say.

I feel the touch of his fingers on the top of my legs. I hear the gentle hiss of the gas fire warming the room. As he moves his hands slowly and carefully I feel vibrations pass up and through me. How does this work? Why do his hands moving gently on my legs make my jaw relax? How little we understand about ourselves and our own bodies – or how little I understand.

I find myself thinking of my ex-husband and how he never touched me like this. How ironic, I think, that a man is touching me the way that almost any woman would enjoy being touched and I'm paying him to learn this. When I was first married I remember wondering why my new husband was only interested in touching my genitals and thinking to myself that there must be men that are interested in kissing their lover's arms. I felt sadness for arms.

'Only the present moment. The last moment is past. Only this moment is real.'

I tried to remember what I was supposed to be thinking and remembered that I wasn't supposed to be thinking at all.

'Be present to the happiness from the touch.'

I tune into the touch and feel contentment, peace, relaxation, gratitude and tenderness – all this, in the present moment, does feel similar to happiness.

'Now, if you'd like to roll over?'

I roll over. I feel so relaxed. Before I started this journey I wouldn't have been able to do this. How many unnecessary inhibitions and insecurities I have lain down. I start thinking about all those who have helped me reach this – T, Hilly, Sue, Justine, Rachael, Nicole, Ken and all those talented men in San Francisco. Thoughts continue to distract from sensation.

He continues his gentle touch, often with one hand holding my hand and another touching my skin. He touches my breasts but doesn't linger on them more than on anywhere else.

As he touches my breasts I think about T and wonder whether the happiness I'm feeling at this stranger's touch is disloyal? But Alexey has a girlfriend too. Is any pleasure that he takes in touching me disloyal? I can hear some of you thinking, 'Yes, it is.' But here is my stance on it – and it's the same with the community at 1080 – the harm is in the lies. If everyone tells the truth there is always choice.

I had an interesting exchange last night with a married man who phoned me. We have had an attraction for many years. He knows, from my Facebook postings, about the OM conference and is curious. He asked me, absolutely sincerely, if he could come over one afternoon and have me teach him how to OM. He said that he'd like to learn from me and I know he meant it. I laughed and then told him, much to his surprise, that it wasn't impossible. 'But you would need to take the OM training with your wife.'

'Oh, she wouldn't be interested in anything like that,' he replied.

'Is that so?' I challenged him right down the phone line. 'Usually when you tell women that OM is a study in female pleasure they are very interested.'

Silence.

'Anyway you could ask her. And if she says yes and you both join the community then, if she's OK with it, you can OM with me as much as you like.'

'But other blokes get to touch her clitoris?'

'Yes. And everyone is honest with everyone. That's my stance. You're welcome as long as no one lies.'

He actually said, 'I wouldn't like any other man touching her. I'm very possessive.' Is this sounding familiar? He'd have come over to my house any afternoon I'd invited him, and been quite happy to deceive his wife. It amazes me what people do to avoid Tolstoy's famous saying, 'The one thing necessary in life, as in art, is to tell the truth.'

'And let that last moment go,' Alexey continued. Oh goodness, what a lot of noise I have in my head.

Then something weird happens. One of those weird woo woo things that I have no explanation for and it sounds as though I'm making it up. But I'm not. He places his hand over my genitals. I think it's the fingers of his right hand, which are facing down as he stands at my right side and holds my right hand with his left hand. And he says something about energy and vibration.

I swear to you I can feel a beam of energy up the inside of my vagina as if someone has switched on a light gun or something.

'What is THAT?' No trouble focusing my energy on this sensation. Wow. It feels like rich deep-red velvet, but made of light. It feels like chocolate. It feels as if the centre of me contains some kind of magnetic force. Now maybe you're all way ahead of me and you've all felt this a million times. But I haven't. Maybe you know that your yoni is an energy field but, although I would have told you that I know that I'm an energy field, I have no experience of feeling a force field inside myself. This is something new.

And then he does another thing I'm not expecting. He leans over and puts his head on my stomach. This feels like

– well, it feels like love. And I'm only saying that it feels, 'like love'. Because I know that you will be sceptical. After all this is a body treatment that I'm paying for. So I don't feel that I can say that it is love – because maybe – just maybe he is a very skilled professional. He is skilled and experienced enough to use real love (which is not so hard to locate) and give unconditionally to all the women that come to him. As Mooji the Advaita teacher says, 'Love loves to love. It's nothing personal.'

Then I remember what he'd said to do. And I take the sensation I'm feeling and breathe and do my best to draw it up to my own heart centre. I do my best to breathe and visualize this.

It's hard not to wrap my arms around him and say, 'Who are you? Where have you been all my life? Can I clone you? I have about a hundred girlfriends that need one of you.'

Then I start to feel the much sought-after waves that I know can rise and become a deep involuntary orgasm. I pounce on the feeling immediately with 100% of my mind demanding, 'Were you a wave? Are you going to grow in intensity? Oh PLEEESE.' I looked around internally hoping for more waves. Unsurprisingly they have vanished from wherever it was they came from.

By this time he has inserted his finger into what is feeling pretty well like some strange force field by now. But instead of massaging it in a purely physical way he's keeping surprisingly still. Just moving a fraction. Each time he moves I feel an unfamiliar vibration, just a little bit of energy going from somewhere to somewhere else. His head is resting on my pubic bone. How strange.

The sensation Isabel – listen to the sensation.

Then another wave. 'Yes! A wave.' I am like someone with a butterfly net – trying to catch an ocean.

Another sensation. Oh no – I need a pee. Damn coffee. Damn tea. This sensation rises quickly. He moves his head slightly.

Inside my head I'm shouting, 'Don't put your head there – I need a pee.' I start to argue with myself.

'Tell him, you stupid woman. He said to say immediately if you need to stop.'

'But it's so beautiful. You can't stop now. Look for waves instead.'

'Yes – focus on the waves.'

'There are no waves.'

'I need to pee.'

Oh, God – now I don't just have noise in my head, I have a debate.

'This feels too good to stop. Maybe that twinge isn't really the bladder – just ride it – maybe you can convert the bladder twinge into a wave.'

'It's hopeless, you just need to pee.'

He moves his head slightly and places it lovingly on my hip bone.

He moves his hand ever so gently. This should feel extraordinary. It does feel extraordinary. But the beam is gone. The waves are gone and the desire to pee is taking over the whole of the lower half of my body. I hate my bladder. It ruins everything.

Five minutes later, I finally speak.

'I'm sorry – I need to pee.'

'A couple more seconds and we're finished. We just have to close.'

'OK, I'll wait,' I say cheerily. As if I'm in a queue outside a public toilet.

Damn, damn. My waves all ruined. My light ray all put out.

He withdraws his finger with infinite gentleness and cups me for a minute or two. Less time, I'm guessing than he would normally. He smiles, 'Go on then. I'll change my clothes.'

I leap up. Have a pee. Put my clothes on and then sit cosily back down on his sofa. He switches off the heater and pours water for us to drink.

I wait for him to say something like, 'So, how was it for you?' But he just waits.

'I had a problem with thoughts in my head.'

'This is a very common problem for women. Men have a higher charge so they find it easier to get out of their heads. It comes with practice. If you are listening to sensation then you can't be in your head. The two cancel each other out.'

'Listening to sensation? That's a good way to describe it. I can do that. I can listen. That's really helpful.'

'What else?' I tell him about the vibrations and the light ray.

'It was very moving when you put your head on my stomach and held me. I wasn't expecting to feel loved here.'

'I did that with a woman once and she immediately started to cry. She told me afterwards that no man had ever held her like that or hugged her in that way. She said she'd had lots of lovers.'

'It makes you wonder, doesn't it?'

'What's wrong with men? Yes, it does,' he said sadly.

I asked about the waves and me leaping on them.

'Often the whole premise of what people practice as sex is about tension. Couples that row a lot, for example, just use sex as a release of tension. This is not the tantric way.'

Hooray. I still maintain that rowing is not part of a healthy relationship.

'I understand that there are two different types of orgasm – the ones that you force and the ones that happen on their own?'

'There are many different types of orgasm. For women, the paradox is that for the best kind to happen you have to forget about it completely. It's not about forcing yourself to deny yourself an orgasm but you learn to make sexual energy so enjoyable in each moment that you don't even look for or care about an orgasm.'

'Being goal-less.' That again.

'Yes. This obsession with irritating the nerve to obtain release from tension is way below what sex can really be. Men need to learn how to love a woman through the body. Women don't need orgasm; they need to feel loved.'

I didn't say, 'And orgasms are nice too.' I just said ...

'Yes.'

'There are men who will do anything for the woman in their lives – they'll work a boring job ten hours a day, they'd give up their lives for her to bring home the money but then they take her to bed at night and just "fuck" her.'

'Not that there is anything wrong with good strong sex, as long as it's not the only thing on the agenda.'

'This here is fun sex and no more than that. It's good for what it's good for – when no more than fun is important to you. For more meaningful sex one has to have love. In our culture no one learns how to love in sex and men simply don't know, practically speaking, how to do it – or even that this is the kind of sex that is good for a woman. I teach both men and women to empower the energy in the yoni and by doing that many healings have taken place.'

'This very old distinction – between making love and having a fuck. I remember a man once said to me, "That expression 'Making love', it's just a stupid soppy expression for 'fucking'." I can hear his words still, echoing down the years. I'd wanted to make love with this man who thought there was only fucking, so it's good to hear you saying the opposite.'

'Of course.'

'So how do you learn to experience the energy that you showed me today?'

'You slow down, become very present inside, listen to the slightest movement and feel your connection as a loving interaction.'

'OK. You know, Alexey, you are a really extraordinary person. There are not many men like you.'

'I'm afraid it's up to women to take the lead in love. It always has been.'

'Yes – well, what I can do – I will do. May I give you a hug?'

'It's a requirement. Yes.' He smiled. I hug him. I put on my boots and I walk out from his eternal evening to the sunny afternoon of an autumn day in North London. And I go home to T to explain everything.

· · ·

Two weeks later and I find myself kicking freshly fallen autumn leaves as I walk down the road toward my second session with Alexey. I don't know where it's all leading but I do know that it's an uncomplicated way to learn.

In a relationship with someone you love there are always difficulties and T and I don't even live together. We don't argue and are never mean or unkind to each other but even with the greatest consideration, his needs, wants and desires are different from mine. How can it not be so in a relationship? I remember a joke about a newly married couple that, spending their first night together, discover that one of them can't sleep with the window open and the other can't sleep with it closed. Some days the difficulties of a relationship feel overwhelming.

As I walk down the hill I'm revising what he told me. I've been practising with T, using the active concept of 'listening to' rather than just 'being aware of' sensation both during OMs and during sex – active 'listening' helps.

I go in and sit down and tell him this immediately.

'The idea you gave me last time, that listening to sensation is a good way to still the noise in the head has been useful. Can you say more about that please?'

'If you are having sex and thinking of other things, it's

as if, while you're with me, I was talking to someone else on the phone. It's having a different conversation. If I'm touching your back and you're thinking about something that happened last week – you're not listening. It's kind of rude.'

'Rude?'

'It's very common and a difficult habit to break sometimes but it's like having another conversation with someone. It's just not relevant.'

'You speak a lot about sexual energy. How would you define it?'

'However you like. It's whatever you want to believe in.'

'What?'

'Some people say that it's simply the hormone system of the body, a physical tension that builds, leads to a swelling of the vaginal lips, etc. But sexual energy certainly seems to be more than just pressing on the nerve.'

'Something is being exchanged other than bodily fluids.'

'Many men don't understand about sexual energy. They watch porn and they try to please women with intensity. I've seen women who have been left bleeding. This man – the last time this happened – was horrified because he was doing what he honestly thought the woman wanted. The "I'm the shit because I can do it so hard and so fast" thinking. I see it all the time.'

We sat in silence for a few minutes.

'Thank God for you, Alexey. The energy that you work with is so gentle and loving. And er, speaking of love – I'm trained not to do projection, but aren't you afraid I'll fall for you a little?'

'Oh, you might do. But you'll find it doesn't matter.'

I laugh at his wise experience.

'And you might fall for me a little?'

'Oh yes, but I fall in love with all the women.'

Ha ha ha ha ha. Oh well, that's OK then.

'Would you like your massage then? And please listen to the sensations. All the sensations. Don't just look out for magic moments, OK?'

I took off my clothes and climbed onto his massage table.

And this time I do manage to shut my mind up and just listen to sensations. They are louder and softer. Thoughts, feelings and sensations rise and fall. When he reaches the yoni, I don't make it any different from the rest of the experience. I'm still listening. He said, 'If the sensations are intense then just breathe them up to your heart,' but I'm not feeling any intense sensations. I notice that some areas seem more receptive to touch than others. Some parts he presses a finger on and it does feel almost numb.

It's not surprising, I tell myself, babies come out of there after all. Then I stop thinking and listen and he touches a different area and a beautiful sensation like a flash of orange passes through me. He's also talking to me sometimes and somehow he creates, or I create (I have no idea which), a strong magnetic pull deep inside me that feels as if it would like to pull him, or him and T, or him and T and the whole planet inside this universe to heal everyone and everything. OK – that sounds a bit dramatic but the best way I can describe a physical sensation with words is to say that it feels like a sensation created to make life well – a deep rich magnetic energy inside a woman.

I was thinking again. There was one place he touched that hurt a little bit and even though he has specifically told me to tell him immediately if anything hurt, I didn't. I just experienced the sensation and had another conversation with myself.

'Ow, that hurts.'

'No, it doesn't.'

'Yes, it does.'

'Are you sure it's not just discomfort?'

'What's the difference between pain and discomfort?'

'Doesn't matter ... it will pass.'

'Ow, it definitely hurts in that area.'

'Then ask him to stop.'

'I'm just feeling the sensation.'

'Did he tell you to just "feel the sensation" if it hurt? No – he didn't. He told you to ask him to stop immediately.'

'OK, he's moved on now. That feels good.'

'Yes, but why didn't you ask him to stop just then?'

'Shut up and listen to the present moment.'

'Now she says this.'

And so on ...

Then slowly back, through images of colour, into sensation. 'That feels a bit like the colour ochre,' then just 'mmmm' and words are gone.

Afterwards, he waits again for me to speak.

'Less noise this time,' I say. Not so much less. A little bit less.

'That's good.'

For some reason I don't tell him about the sensation of pain or that I didn't stop him. I feel stupid. He's doing everything to please me. I'm experiencing discomfort and saying nothing. Honestly – don't you feel sorry for men everywhere? How common is this? I just decide that I'll take a note myself and never do this again.

I have never done this with T. In the almost one year that I've now been with T, I have experienced some discomfort maybe twice and said 'Ow' and instantly he's stopped. I know how to do this. Maybe it's because of everything I've heard about the need for vaginal massage to be painful – as if something can be released in this way. Am I brainwashed? But it was maybe a second or two of the entire experience. The massage as a whole was, well ...

'It was beautiful, Alexey. I can see how strong my habit of not listening fully is.'

'Yes, you need to learn to listen for the most subtle of sensations.'

'I'm incredibly moved by your gentleness – it doesn't feel like yoni massage at all. Or not as I've known it. It feels more like love.'

'Anything to do with the yoni is about love. That's the energy of the yoni in a woman.'

'It's incredible how just you resting your hand on the outside seems to create a feeling like a deep well. A magnetic field in the base of me.'

I don't feel this with T. I'm too focused on him and his sensation. But here I am forced to understand that it isn't about Alexey so no such cop out is available.

'I can't say it often enough to women or men. It's about listening to the most subtle sensations. Not dismissing them but enjoying them.'

'Yes. I can see that, even in OMing, which they describe as a goal-less practice, I've ended up wanting more. I know in every other area of my life that less is more. I don't want a larger house, or larger car or a more expensive handbag. I know this in every other area so why have I forgotten it in sexuality?'

'It's something that it seems everyone has forgotten. I'm always hearing that people just want "sensational sex" and they want it every time.'

'But we don't always want art that is glaring or music that is deafening. We enjoy subtlety in other areas of life?'

'The nuances have become overlooked in sex. It's more variation on the bigger, harder, faster, "more more more" school of thought.'

'Porn to blame again?'

'Yes. I ask what's wrong with sensational sex SOMETIMES and subtle, gentle sex on others? Even bad sex sometimes. That could be OK too.'

'Yeh, nothing wrong with pizza sometimes. We have been brainwashed into thinking that we want a feast every time.'

'Somehow. Yes.'

I hope this is obvious to you. I hope you haven't been aiming at 'sensational sex'. But I suppose even the premise of this book – which is about making sex as good as we can make it in our relationships – means that we want a different definition of 'good'. Good doesn't mean 'red hot' every day. Good means sometimes light blue sex with a little green. Maybe orange. Sometimes the sensation maybe a far-off yellow like a distant sunrise that turns to a glowing light orange and then subsides into sleepy velvet night. Sometimes maybe even white. Think of the infinite variety of art, of music, of flavour.

'Surely good sex can be more varied than art or music or great foods?'

'Yes, much more.'

'Goodness Alexey, I want so much less. And women can feel more with less stimulation?'

'Sometimes, yes. Often, when people are training their hearing,' Alexey says, 'they have to learn how to hear quieter and quieter sounds. It's like that.'

I want to rush home and say to T. 'Move less or better still – don't move at all.'

'So, are there lots of couples out there who, because they are not having "sensational sex", end up having no sex because they think that it isn't working?'

'Yes. That's it exactly.'

• • •

Later that evening T joins me for dinner. He's been listening to a friend of his complaining that, 'Having kids can kill a couple's sex life for years.'

Fresh from listening to Alexey we discuss this and why it need not be so. What his friend who had made this complaint had meant is, 'having kids leaves you no energy or time for all-singing, all-dancing "sensational" sex where huge red fireworks are going off.' Because of course the fact that one partner could put a hand on the other partner's skin and send an energetic vibration through them that would feel a little bit like the colour yellow – wouldn't count. Because noticing that if you rub your finger on someone's lips it can produce a great feeling in your feet – that doesn't count. What this couple, whoever they were, had decided was – it had to be pillar-box red or nothing.

'What about white, T?'

'What?'

And I told him about the other colours.

'Doesn't a definition of good sex include all the colours?'

'Yes. And I think you're right. He's forgotten this. I've forgotten it too.'

We went back to T's house and nuzzled into his bed for a night of light orange and ochre sex with a sprinkling of blue and a little white.

The Love, Sex and Intimacy Weekend Fair

One of the wonderful things about exploring sexuality is that there is always more to learn, more bizarre opportunities. Thankfully, interest in what makes sex work well seems to be on the increase. This autumn, I'm invited to speak at a 'Love, Sex and Intimacy Fair' in Brighton. Well, Hove actually. This is a very good excuse for T and me to visit friends and attend interesting events. You just never know what you're going to learn.

We arrive on the Saturday morning and, more by luck than good judgement, walk straight into a 'hands-on' workshop led by a lusciously curvaceous Rachael McCoy. Rachael is a young mum who has been working with sex toys and teaching workshops of various kinds for seven years. She'll come to your home and do this event for you and your friends if you ask her nicely.[19] She is like a queen wearing a gorgeous red dress and presenting to us in a crimson 'tantric tent' that the organizers had created specially with beautiful hangings, rugs and cushions in deep reds and golds. There are about 40 of us piled in; a good gender balance and mostly couples. This is a participatory workshop called 'Techniques for Him and Techniques for Her'. But – thank God – everyone is keeping their clothes on.

Rachael gives every woman in the room a life-size 'erect penis and scrotum' set made of something rubbery and every man a rubber model with clitoris, vulva with inner and outer lips and vaginal opening, perineum (or 'geish' as it's defined in the Urban Dictionary) and anus. The models look and feel alarmingly lifelike. T has bagged two places at the front.

'Could you all wipe your hands with a medi-wipe? We are going to be touching toys and this is to protect the toys from any dirt that may be on your hands.'

We clean our hands conscientiously.

'Let's start with a tip for the women,' she says while handing round some tubes of lube, all the better to slide with on the demo toy.

'I'm sure you women are already very good at giving men

pleasure with your hands ...' she says cheerfully, 'but here is a new tip to try. The most sensitive part of the man's penis is the "frenulum".' This much I know, although men friends have said that there is no wrong part to stroke. 'One of the variations on the classic "corkscrew movement" of the hand ...' she says, holding up the lubed penis and rubbing her red nail-varnished hands over the head repeatedly 'is to change to just using your thumb and second finger and to grip quite firmly. If you would all like to try that ladies?' She says as if she's telling us how to apply lipstick.

'Would anyone like any more lube?'

A couple of men in the tent remove their jackets.

'When you are pleasing your man in this way be sure to be in his eyeshot. Bend over and move your body in a sensual way to add to his pleasure as men are very visual.' She demonstrates this while continuing to move between the 'corkscrew' and the 'two-finger' pleasuring method.

T seems to be looking a little flushed. I see him smile at me.

'And now for the men,' she says, picking up one of the 'women' genital models.

'Men, when you are pleasuring a woman, it's very important not to dive straight between her legs. Women don't like this. If you want to give a woman pleasure, it's good to start with a massage that may be a movement like this that slides your hands down her stomach and onto the inside of her legs. You can also use your whole body.'

'Can someone help me demo this?'

I volunteer. 'And your name is?'

'Isabel.'

'OK Isabel, could you lie down on these pillows?' I oblige. 'So, men, you would start this massage here on her stomach and then go round her hips and then down her legs. You could keep doing this until she asks you to move to the outer lips.' She rubs her hands down the inside of my legs and then up over the calves. 'OK Isabel, you can sit up now. Could you hold the model?'

I hold up the rubber genitals. 'It's a good warm-up to slide all your four fingers over the entire area in a sweeping motion like this.' She slides her whole hand down in an 'S' shape. 'And then up again with a gentle pushing.' She makes a figure of eight. 'There is no direct stimulation of the clitoris but this feels very good for the woman. After this you can use your whole body.'

Men run their fingers over the models while women smile and watch Rachael performing so brilliantly on women's behalf.

'Thank you, Isabel.'

I return to my place obediently. 'Now – another tip for the women. You're going to practise a fast hand stimulation of the penis in an up-and-down movement along with slow stroking of the scrotum. Women are often a little afraid of the balls and confused by them because it seems to women that on the one hand they can be quite easily hurt, while during intercourse they can be banging around quite firmly and the man isn't in any pain. So it's good to talk to your man about this and find out what is pleasurable for him.'

'Could you hold the model, please?' T gets up and holds

the erect penis against his chest while she demonstrates a fast speed with one hand and slow stroking with the other. 'You can even use your nails gently against his scrotum as many men like this.' T removes his shirt and only has a tight-fitting black T-shirt left. I wonder if that's coming off next.

'You may like to take your T-shirt off so it doesn't get any lube on it.'

T obediently removes his T-shirt, so is now holding the erect penis against his skin. His weekends this year are rarely predictable.

'Yes, that's very good.' Rachael looks around the tent approvingly. When you are pleasuring a man with your hands remember you have the option to vary three things: speed, pressure and rhythm. With this movement it may help you to have some kind of music in your head so you have one rhythm for the base stroke and one for the upper stroke.'

'Thank you.' T sits down and takes out his water bottle. 'Another one for the men,' she says. The men all lube up again. She shows them how they can move from a sensual rub over the vagina to gently pushing the middle finger forward and entering the woman with one finger or two.

'Always keep the channels of communication open,' she says, 'so that the woman can tell you what she enjoys and what she would like more of. Some women like just one finger gently and some women enjoy more than one finger – you really need to find out how to please your woman. Never assume that something pleases her.'

'Now – for the women – about anal stimulation ...' She

chatters on.

'Anal stimulation is extremely pleasurable for men – especially if you stimulate the prostate, which is between one-and-a-half and three inches inside the anal canal.'

I raise my hand and ask, 'I've heard that prostate massage helps prevent prostate cancer?'

'I've heard this too but I don't talk about that as I'm not trained medically. We are just concentrating on pleasure here.'

'OK.'

'So, before you begin this, if you worry about faeces then it's usual to use an anal douche.' She holds one up. 'You simply fill it with warm water and douche out the contents to be sure you're clean. They are easy to get used to.'

Obviously we've all used an anal douche then? Have I lived a very tame life?

'Women, if you put your finger an inch or two down the anal canal you will find a round bulb of tissue – this is the prostate and you massage it using a "come here" motion with your finger.'

I contemplate all this uncertainly. I've massaged lovers externally and played around a bit with a finger or two but never attempted a real and focused prostate massage.

T leans over and whispers, 'I once endured this "treatment" from a male doctor when my prostate was inflamed. It was complete agony.'

'Perhaps it wouldn't be agony if it wasn't inflamed,' I whisper back.

Rachael continues her talk as if she were discussing garden flowers. 'This kind of massage is likely to give a man a more intense orgasm than he is likely to have experienced through penetration.'

'Do you want to try?' I whisper to T.

'I'm not sure – maybe.'

'One last thing I'd like to talk about,' she smiles. 'Smacking.'

'If one of you would like to bend over? I need a volunteer. You again, sir.' She points at T.

'Do I have to take my clothes off?' he asks, perhaps a little eagerly.

'No – sorry. But bend over.' She bends him over her knee. 'Ladies – there are different ways to smack depending on what kind of pain you'd like to produce. Obviously, none of this pain is severe – but it can sting a bit and lots of couples like it as a warm-up. You can slap using the full flat of your hand like this.' She slaps him cheerfully. 'Or you can cup your hand and slap him like this ...'

Slap. Slap.

And what did you feel, Isabel, to see her slapping your boyfriend's butt? Well, he's clothed, so I think it's fun. I can't see T's face so I'm not sure whether he's enjoying it or not, but I'm guessing he is. And even if he isn't – it's another experience.

'Now – the other way around.'

'Men, if you bend your women over?' There were no chairs so we were all standing at this point. I bend over and get slapped. My inner child isn't too happy about this. 'But I haven't done anything naughty,' I complain. 'Oh, I'm sure you must have done something bad,' he smiles. Slap.

It doesn't really hurt but it's decidedly undignified. Oh, for heaven's sake, I used to get up to these antics when I was 19 – along with dressing up in my school uniform for my then boyfriend's enjoyment. But I feel a little bit beyond all this now.

'How do you feel about slapping?' T asks me.

'There are other things I'd rather try.'

'That's OK – we don't have to like all of this.'

'One final demo that works for men or women,' Rachael says. 'If you are going to demo this one you'll have to take your T-shirt off again,' she says to T.

I had promised this man, when he started this, that the experience may involve many emotions but that boredom would never be one of them. It appears I'm keeping my word.

'Oh, if you insist,' he says, stripping to his jeans.

'I just don't want to get lube on your clothes. If you could lie down here?'

It's generous of T to sacrifice himself for us all, isn't it?

'If your partner is orgasmic ...' she says to us as she steps over him, '... if he has come it feels really good if you massage him afterwards, like this.' She runs her flattened hands up from the top of his trousers and down over his arms. 'It helps your lover take the energy and integrate it into his entire body more.'

T lies with his eyes closed, grinning. I can see that postcoital massage is going to be on his request list from now on.

'And it will be a more complete experience for a woman

if you give her this kind of attention, men. Instead of falling asleep.'

OK – and mine too.

'And that's "Techniques for Him and Techniques for Her".'

We all applaud with genuine admiration. What a sparky, gutsy, sexy, sassy lady Rachael is.

'If we get together a group of couples, could you visit a home to do this demo?' asks T. 'Yes – just visit my website.'

T puts his clothes on again. Everyone is surprisingly clothed at this fair.

The next session we choose is about 'Getting Intimate with Your Beloved'. I'd thought it might be good for us to attend as it may help to address some of the difficulties we are experiencing in our relationship. But when we get there it's like 'Relating 101' – the first process is about looking into each other's eyes. There's nothing wrong with what they're teaching – it's the pace at which they're teaching. And the voice. I could hear my daughter in my ear saying, 'Oh God, it's the Mystic Meg voice.' You know when people in the spiritual or tantra world speak as if everyone was a client? 'How does this make you FEEL?' [pause before the F-word to add an inappropriate level of stress to anything to do with emotion]. Then they tell us how, if you find yourself in a 'bad place' with your partner you can ask to 'express an appreciation'. Again, it's a lovely concept but I whispered in T's ear, 'If you can ever see that I'm in a bad mood and you ask whether you can "express an appreciation", I must warn you that you may be told to fuck off.'

'Why not just say something nice rather than ask if you

can "express an appreciation" first?' he whispers to me.

'It's supposed to be respectful.'

After we'd done some looking into each other's eyes and repeating, 'Something I love about you is ...' about 20 times each, they move on to creating a 'special time' for yourselves. We find a moment when people are moving about to grab our shoes, escape the tent and go and explore *The Great Wall of Vagina*.

The artist Jamie McCartney has made a wall of plaster casts of women's vulvas and a number of the pieces are being exhibited here. Rows and rows of what women look like between the legs, in plaster. Punters are staring. I know I've spoken about this before but women simply have no idea what other women look like and many women don't even know what they look like themselves. We are all surprised by the variety and Jamie confirms this.

'Every woman is amazed when she sees the wall,' he says. 'Women of all ages and sizes think that they are different from normal but, as you see here, there is no normal. Every woman is "normal".'

'I never knew inner lips could be that big,' says a woman pointing at one cast.

'I didn't know outer lips could be that big,' the man beside her points at another.

Meanwhile a mother is here with her little girl – who must be aged about eight. They're looking at the wall and talking about them all. 'I wish I'd seen this when I was that age,' I say to Jamie. 'Then I'd have known all my life that I was normal instead of thinking there was something a bit odd about my shape.'

'I've heard this from so many women,' Jamie said. 'Which of these is the most "normal" do you think?'

'The one there with very little inner lips?'

'But most women have protruding inner lips.'

'I can see that.'

Since T and I have been OMing he could probably match mine to one more closely than I could.

'I think this work is fantastic, Jamie. And beautiful. It deserves a special exhibition at Tate Modern. This work is important. This could save some women from having unnecessary operations. Why aren't you at the Tate?'

'You have to be invited, Isabel. No one's invited me.'

'Well, they should have.'

It takes a while to shift my brain from 'that one's weird' to 'this shows variations on a part of the human body'. If they were faces everyone would see beauty, but after looking for a while I see beauty here too. I think I know lots of people who couldn't look at this art though. Art that challenges the way I see and alters my perceptions.

I'm really impressed. Weird, huh? If you want to look for yourself or have a cast made of your own vulva lips for a lover – you can arrange this with Jamie and he'll make you one.[20] You weren't expecting that Christmas gift suggestion were you?

In the evening, my ego's delighted to have a full house for my own talk. I'm speaking about one of my previous books, *Men!* This book addresses the well-known sociological phenomenon that we all know many single women but have very few single male friends to introduce them to. Many women mix in social circles that are exclusively female and feel lonely not only for lovers but for brothers and even male friends. I explain to my audience how and why this has happened. It's a fun presentation that I did for a year and I always enjoy a live audience and the privilege of making people laugh. I also tell them what I didn't know when I wrote that book but which I know now. One place where men will always be found is in any event, seminar or workshop in the positive sex or conscious sex movement. Even the audience I address there, for perhaps the first time in my career, is 50% male. So women readers, if you want to find lovers, go to anywhere that looks at taking responsibility for your sexuality. You'll find men there.

• • •

On Sunday morning, I escape the book stall with only a British Museum book *Haiku on Love*; weave my way carefully past the 'Raw Chocolate' stall'[21] and sample the raw ginger, coconut, orange and cardamom chocolate; breathe in the gorgeous scents of Haskel Adamson's Neroli and Rose women's massage oil[22] (and buy that for me and Sandalwood and Vetiver men's massage oil for T) before joining T for coffee.

We sit and look at the people there. It's mainly an alternative crowd. Some of the people who are offering body-painting, permanent make-up or fetish clothing are displaying the products themselves. But there's also a range of more everyday-looking singles and couples aged from their early 20s to early 70s that are sitting around chatting.

A couple of girls who are friends of friends come up and say hello. We compare notes.

'What's everyone going to next?' T browses the various speakers.

'I like the sound of this talk,' says a woman in bright red shoes with heels that must be about 12 inches high. It's a spectator sport just seeing her walking in them but she's certainly getting attention. 'There is a lady called Nic Ramsey who runs the She Said Erotic Boutique giving a talk called "The Ultimate Sex Secret Every Woman Should Know".'

'I'd like to know it,' says her friend. 'I haven't had sex in a year – I want to know all the secrets I can.'

We agree on this.

'But let's try and guess,' I suggest. 'What do you each think the secret will be? If you were giving a talk with that name what would you talk about?'

'I'd talk about how every woman is different,' says one woman.

'And so?' I ask.

'So, it's important for men to take things slowly and find out what works for her. I would talk about women with vaginismus[23] and how empowering it can be to discover sex from a female perspective rather than a male one.'

'My talk would be called "Make Love not Porn".' says a smiling face called Erin.

'Mine would be called "No Fear – Embrace What You Both Like",' says a face called Lizzie.

'But what do you think "The Ultimate Sex Secret" is?' I ask.

'That it's good to be a little selfish,' suggests a third face called Pamela.

Then a man speaks: 'Learn to be in touch with your own body before you can expect a man to do the same.' We look around.

'What about you, Isabel? What do you think's the ultimate sexual secret that every woman should know?'

'I really have no idea. If it's a secret, I probably don't know it.'

We finish our drinks and go off to the tantra tent for the talk. I'd guess that Nic's in her mid-40s – a sassy petite blonde. After she has us all settled comfortably she introduces herself briefly.

'People always ask how I ended up running a sex shop. And they're always surprised with my reply. After moving to Brighton in 2000, my then fiancé broke my heart, calling off our wedding four weeks before the big day, saying that I was "frigid". And the truth was, he was right. After years of gynaecological problems resulting in a bad body image and just not enjoying sex, I decided I had to face my demons and learn about sex. So I opened a sex shop. As you do. One aimed at women.'

We applauded. She bowed and continued,

'Fifteen years on, I can safely say that my heartbreak turned out to be the best thing that ever happened to me. There isn't a single day when I don't make a change in at least one person's life by sharing my knowledge and helping women to feel better about themselves, their bodies and their sexuality.'

I can't imagine running a sex shop. Her days must be infinitely varied.

'The title of this talk is designed to draw you in, and I see that it has done so very successfully. And of course there is not one secret – there are many. But I'm going to talk to you today about a secret that few women understand fully – the influence on our health and our sex lives of ... drum roll ... pelvic floor muscles.'

No one had predicted that, but Nic knows her subject, so women – listen up.

I'd be willing to bet that you've all underestimated the importance of having healthy and strong pelvic floor muscles. You don't need toys to exercise them but Nic's erotica boutique, as well as selling 'all kinds of fun things',[24] takes these muscle toys seriously. She has 'Luna beads', which may not be jade eggs but they are a damn sight better than the dog-toy-style appliance that Jovanna had mocked me for purchasing. There are even pressure pumps on her site that measure the strength of the pelvic floor and a metal weight, a sample of which she passes round.

'There are women who can lift something this heavy?' someone asks.

Yes, apparently there are.

'One good exercise is to imagine that you have a marker pen in your vagina and are trying to write your name with it. This will get you to contract your muscles in all kinds of new ways.'

'Have you tried it?' asked a voice from the back.

'Not yet. But maybe I will. First of all, the muscles have to be strong enough to hold the pen in place.' I look forward to receiving your pictures.

As I've been reading extensively this year I understand, but I notice with interest how little the other women know. Nic tells one story that is shocking – it may not be true but I wouldn't be surprised. Apparently one of the bestselling products in our high street chemists is incontinence pads for adult women. The story Nic reports is that one of the better-known chains started to sell pelvic floor muscle exercisers – but someone noticed that the more of these they sold the fewer incontinence pads were bought in that town. Bearing in mind that the pads of all kinds are such a bestselling product, what did they do? Advertise the exercisers to benefit more women? No, you've guessed, haven't you? They stopped selling the pelvic exercisers to keep profit in pads high. I don't make these stories up and I haven't verified this but it seems possible. Having asked a few quick questions of women on my Facebook pages, so many admit 'avoiding trampolines and coughing'. I'm really surprised that these exercises are not more widely talked about. And do they really improve our sex lives? Surely if this claim is also true then let's do our bit to put the makers of incontinence pads out of business. Or at any rate, let's ensure that neither you nor any of the women you know are contributing to those profits.

The Love, Sex and Intimacy Fair was drawing to a close. T and I decide to skip the last workshop to take the train from Hove Actually back to London. People leaving are sporting leather trousers, whips and fetish paraphernalia. We have massage oil and a book from the British Museum. On the train I'm seized with a moment of doubt.

'You don't want to whip me do you, T? You don't wish I dressed in rubber and want to put a chain around your neck? I'm not the most boring woman in the UK, am I?'

'No darling, you're not. And this has not been a dull weekend.' He produced a box of the amazing orange and cardamom chocolate from the Sexy Raw Chocolate stall. And as we share it and I doze on his shoulder on the way home I know why I'm doing all this. It isn't all about sex is it?

Your 'Sex Muscles' – Kegels and the NHS

So – if strong pelvic floor muscles can really improve our sex lives then I must research this immediately. To do so I must digress to tell you a story. It is a true story and one in which I believe you may have the greatest interest.

There was once a woman who went down in history with the name of Mary Cool. This is not her real name but is the name that her case study was given. She was a US citizen and 42 years old. She had been married for 20 years. She and her husband had sex twice a year.

At the age of 42 Mary started to suffer from a problem which affects more and more women from an increasingly early age – incontinence. Whenever she sneezed, coughed or lifted a weight urine would leak and sometimes drench her. Apparently one out of every two women suffer from this problem at some point in their lives. Mary suffered this embarrassing situation for seven years before going to the doctor who recommended an operation.

Now, as it happens sometimes, Mary had a friend who was into weird alternative stuff. The friend was not afraid to give a little unsolicited advice.

'Look here,' she said ...

Ha – I'm making this up of course. I have no idea what conversation took place at this point in the story.

'Mary, you don't have to have an operation.'

'But the doctor said ...' blubbed Mary, sobbing, coughing and wetting her pants again.

'Just listen to me,' said the well-meaning and interfering friend.

'I know a different doctor. He's called Arnold Kegel. And he has a non-surgical method to cure you.'

'Oh, sure, and does he believe in fairies too?' sniffed Mary.

'It works like this,' persevered the woo woo friend. 'You have to work hard but you need to rehabilitate the muscles that have collapsed, which is why you have the problem that you have. It's the muscles that hold up the whole of your insides. It's actually a ring of muscles.'

'But mine are damaged beyond repair,' she sobbed damply.

'No. Dr Kegel has this thingamajig that he calls a perineometer. It gets inserted into the vagina and you have to squeeze it.'

'But I won't be able to. Nothing in that part of my body works.'

'Just go and see him, OK? You may avoid the operation.'

So our Mary went along to see the now very famous Dr Kegel. His thingamajig did indeed show that the pelvic floor was totally distended. We could be mean and say atrophied. When she tried to squeeze, the machine measured zero pressure. She was not in a good way. But, keen as we all would be to avoid an operation, Mary went away and practised.

After only six weeks of her daily pelvic floor muscles workout she was able to squeeze and a score of 12mm (whatever that is) showed on the perineometer.

Six months later she was cured and was able to cancel the intended operation. By the time the story ends Mary was squeezing the perineometer and the machine was measuring a score of 22mm. The medical records also inform us that 'her vaginal muscles became much thicker and stronger'.

But here's the bit of the story that should really get your attention. About Mary's sex life. In her bi-annual sexual encounters Mary had reported no sensation and certainly never had a climax of any kind. Now she told Dr Kegel that she wished she had known 20 years ago that it was possible to train these muscles. She was now having sex with her much happier husband several times a week and had experienced her first climax.

She and her friend went out and bought expensive silk lingerie to celebrate.

OK, so I hope it's clear which bits of this story are me playing and which bits are historically accurate. This case is recorded in 1951 and is one of those that made Dr Kegel famous. In hundreds of further cases he established a link between lack of sexual response and distended Kegel muscles. Also, the other way around. Women who reported being very sexually responsive were shown to have very strong and elastic Kegel muscles. The people in this last group never suffer from incontinence and have few gynaecological problems.

It works like this – the vaginal muscles are sensitive because they are full of nerves. But the mucous membrane of the vagina has very few nerve endings and is almost insensitive. Distension of the muscles therefore renders them less sensitive. And what distends them? Childbirth, being overweight, constipation, lack of exercise, infrequent sex, and general bad health. And after menopause the muscles will thin anyway, but only if they are not used.

But the news is good, girls. Using these muscles regularly restores the functions of the vaginal glands and these are the glands that secrete female hormones as well. Andre Van Lysebeth, from whose book I have taken the retelling of this case history, even goes as far as to say that he believes this practice helps to prevent osteoporosis.

The benefits of strengthening the pelvic floor muscles for men include curing incontinence and improving muscle tone, which can help delay ejaculation. Some sources even say that exercising these muscles can massage and relax the prostate, which may help to prevent prostate cancer. Apparently six months' pelvic floor muscles training for men is more effective than Viagra in reversing erectile dysfunction. In short, getting blood to these bits is good for all of us.

But back to Mary. What I really want you to notice

about the story is that Mary required not one single other experience to improve her sex life from twice a year to twice a week. No one asked about her sexual history, no one offered her yoni healing and, as far as the records show, she may not even have known the location of her clitoris. This was the US in 1951 after all. She hadn't been to see Freud or Jung, and I think we can safely assume that she had never read a book on tantra. Now I'm not saying that everything I've written about so far is null and void – of course not – it all goes together. And, you can call me Isabel Cool if you like, but I intend to follow Mary's journey and report back to you.

• • •

You may be amazed to know that a lot of help is available to you on the NHS if you'd like to tone up your pelvic floor. You don't have to be sick. You don't have to be incontinent. I thank goodness I'm not. But quite what state my pelvic floor muscles are in remains to be seen. I go to see my doctor and explain that, for a number of reasons, I'm interested in checking the health of my pelvic muscles and does she know anyone with a perineometer? She says that if I want to check whether they're OK, I've purely to see whether I can stop peeing mid-flow. But she refers me anyway to a delightful uro-gynae nurse, as an outpatient at my local hospital.

Now before you raise your eyebrows and think this is a questionable use of NHS resources, in this case it's quite legitimate. There are people in the NHS whose job it is to improve the quality of life. You don't have to be sick to go and see a doctor. The uro-gynae nurse sighs when I repeat my

GP's comment and says, 'We don't use that stopping mid-flow test any more.' She's a wonderfully positive woman who tells me, 'I wanted to be a nurse but I didn't want to work with sick people. I love this job because it genuinely improves the quality of people's lives.' She explains that I need to come back and see a 'pelvic floor physiotherapist' and that, surprisingly, the waiting list isn't long. I could have just researched the exercises at home but I'm curious to know just how bad or good a state my pelvic floor muscles are in. I am trying to represent the majority of women out there – and, assuming that the majority of women are not incontinent which is the point at which most women go to their doctor – find out just how poor a state these muscles may be in.

May I assume you know about them? Most men and women do. I was told about them after I'd given birth to my daughter (not before – which would have been wise) and I've practised them a bit over the years but not with any discipline. In France it's standard practice for women to be given help re-training these muscles after birth, but not in the UK or the US. I've run regularly for cardiovascular health and, yes, that's probably good. But Kegel muscles? Well, does anyone exercise them regularly?

So while I wait for my NHS appointment to come up – long live the NHS – I do a little research on what can be done if your local GP is less helpful than mine or your local hospital does not boast a team of pelvic floor physiotherapists.

Some women don't even know what Kegel muscles or pelvic floor muscles are. I discover this by asking the 3,000 people that follow my Facebook pages. I just ask how often people exercise them. Answers include,

'I don't know what you are talking about – never heard of them.'

'Never done them.'

'... whenever I pee – in a start-stop action.' (This is not recommended any more as I told you.)

'Whenever I have sex.' (This is better but she added, 'This isn't very often.')

Or, 'Only when I'm reminded of them by reading a question like this.'

And, 'Used to do them all the time and now can't be bothered and, erm, notice the difference. Cough, cough ... oops.'

The best answer, 'once or twice a week for about 45 seconds'.

And one women friend says, 'I always do them on "up" escalators'.

Bearing in mind the low levels of orgasmic response in women and the large numbers that suffer incontinence, some from having their first child in their early 20s, these responses are worrying. It is recognized that for both women and men a wide range of health problems can be avoided by not having any part of the bottom half of your body going into prolapse.

I suppose that, perhaps inevitably, there is also some information on the Internet saying the opposite – on the dangers of too much Kegel exercise. But, firstly, they seem to be coming from only one source and, secondly, from my brief and unscientific survey, it seems that there is very little danger of anyone doing too many exercises of this kind.

So – which are your pelvic floor muscles? If you do a quick Internet search pictures will appear of the underside of both men and women and you can read up and become knowledgeable. For our purposes and, very simply, they circle the urethra, the vagina and the anal canal.

The problem with exercising these muscles is that it's not very interesting. Even when recommended by a doctor, compliance with a pelvic floor exercise programme is poor. If you don't want to go to your GP, there is a range of fun toys to play with at home. You could check out 'Kegel 8'. But I would get the biofeedback pelvic trainer, not the machine that does the exercises for you while you watch TV. Call me narrow-minded but I just don't believe that electronically stimulating a muscle so that it contracts is the same as actually contracting it yourself.

Let me tell you some of the ways to enjoy these exercises. The first is a weird one as you wouldn't expect it to be enjoyable – but strangely it is. Try and suck your anus up into your body. To really lift it. The muscle that you are using is called your *levator ani*. Yes, your 'lift anus' muscle. Just go on and on lifting that muscle slowly and firmly and you may feel a vibration and even a shiver go up your spine. Weird, huh? You could hold it for up to ten seconds and then release. As Andre Van Lysebeth tells us, 'a pleasant feeling of warmth is felt at the base of the body in the lumbar region'. You can also practise lifting the anus up as high as you can while breathing normally.

This exercise is a good way to never be bored again while

sitting down. Any waiting for a bus or a train, a plane or a person and you can entertain yourself with this one. I'm sorry to be personal but if you have even one haemorrhoid – perhaps following childbirth if you are a woman, or spending too long reading in the loo if you're a man – and you do this exercise, do please drop me a line and let me know how long you practised for and whether the problem lifted itself away.

As I said, the muscles form loops around our various openings so by doing this exercise you are also drawing your awareness to the muscles between the anus and the vulva, perineum, the uterus and even the clitoris. Getting a little extra blood to these parts is very good for us.

• • •

Women – I keep hearing again and again, from a wide range of sources, that if you have a vibrator it's a good idea not to switch it on. Really. Everyone I've met and spoken to in the positive sexuality world agrees on this. This may strike you as odd as I've said that stimulating the nerves can be good if you are doing it yourself but artificially overstimulating the nerves makes them go dead. After a while, women simply can't feel anything. Please don't write and tell me this is nonsense – I'm just telling you what I've heard from everyone that works in this discipline. Even a woman who sells vibes told me this.

One day T and I went to visit a well-known independent sex shop and while we were there we struck up a conversation with the woman that ran the shop. We asked her about this. 'It's true,' she said. 'That's why women are always coming in here and asking for something stronger. They want them stronger and stronger. I never use them myself.' Should we be concerned about the vibe sales in the increasing number of sex shops across the country? They may be numbing our pleasure rather than increasing it. They are certainly not designed to help you listen for the subtle.

There is one exception. The vibe is fine as long as you take the batteries out – recycle them – and use it for strengthening your Kegel muscles. But you'd better only do this exercise if you've put the batteries a long way away. You can have fun without them. Really. So in order to strengthen the vaginal muscles we need to widen them first. In order to constrict a sphincter you have to widen it first. So, carefully lubricate and insert the vibe, grasp as firmly as you can and hold for a few seconds, then relax the muscle fully. This is a good one for listening to as many sensations as you can, however subtle. If you place your awareness there you will increasingly become aware of more subtle sensations. You can breathe in – do the lifting – and breathe out. There are lots of variations. If you really want to become an expert, see if you can make circular motions with the vibe. The possibilities are endless.

Another exercise much praised by the tantric masters is the ability to contract the muscle at the opening and work the muscles upwards all the way to the cervix and then down again. To learn this – I'm told – you first constrict the entire vagina and then learn to relax them one bit at a time until it becomes easy and produces a wave-like motion inside the vagina. A real tantric mistress would know how to mimic the spontaneous undulating motions that occur during an orgasm for her partner's pleasure. I look forward to your letters on this section.

And it's like learning to play any other instrument – daily, short practice sessions are better than twice a week longer ones. It's less fun without a vibe but of course you can practise these on the bus or the tube. If you spot a woman reading this book on a bus with a strangely ecstatic look on her face you know what she's doing.

And about dance classes. I'm always telling women that if you want to meet men, don't go to 'hips, bums and tums', yoga or any dance class that is 98% female. Go climbing, go learn how to row, learn scuba diving – anything that will have at least a 50% male attendance. But – if you must go to an all-female dance class – why not try belly dancing? Pelvic mobility is the way to go. Tilt the sex organs up and down and this way and that way. Thrust the pelvis, rotate the pelvis, twirl the pelvis in a sexually provocative way ... yes, yes, it's yet one more way of exercising that all-important area of your body.

• • •

So, a week later I find myself being examined by a specialist pelvic floor physiotherapist at my local hospital. They have a team and they see women of all ages. It's important to have these muscles healthy before childbirth, after childbirth and, well, for anyone that has a bladder – before you even consider your sex life.

My nurse, Clare, is very matter of a fact about it all. But, there's no machine. I'm disappointed. 'I thought you had a machine to tell women how good or bad their pelvic floor strength is.'

'No, we prefer a trained specialist to a machine. It's possible to cheat with a machine because, for example, you can get a reading using your abs or your inner thigh muscles – whereas I can tell which muscles you are using much better with my fingers.'

More women's fingers up my vagina. Sigh. I'm almost getting used to it.

'I see.' Is this going to be better or worse than the colonic examination I told you about in *The Battersea Park Road to Enlightenment?*

'We have a simple way of describing the muscles that you need to use. For the back muscles you imagine that you have a fart that you don't want to release. So I say, "hold wind". Then for the front muscles you imagine that your bladder is full but you can't get to a toilet. That is, lift the *pube rectalis*, or "hold wee".

'The pube erectalis?'

'No, *rectalis*. The *levitor ani*.'

'OK.'

'Then I'm going to ask you to hold the muscle for a count of ten not using any of your other muscles to hold the contraction. It's important to relax the muscle fully after that.'

'OK.'

'So I'm going to put my finger inside you now, OK?'

Sigh. I've said this before – thank God this isn't television.

'OK, so now, "hold wind". And, "hold wee". And firmer.

Think of pulling the anus up and the squeezing my fingers forward ... 5, 6, 7, 8 ...'

Honestly, my dedication knows no limits. And people worry about having their 'personal details' on Facebook?

'... and 10. Very good. That was a good relaxation. So if you do that exercise where you draw the muscles up and hold for a count of ten – ten times, five times a day. Here is the second exercise. Just pull the muscles right up and then release, as firmly as you can ... let's see how many you can do, OK?'

I'm determined to impress her and go past ten strong squeezes.

'OK, so let's see if you can get to 20?'

'Shouldn't I be able to keep going indefinitely?' I asked, attempting not to screw my face up to help.

'Not really. You see they are getting weaker. And keep going ... 18, 19 and ... 20.'

'Very good. So practise that exercise five times a day too. We'll see you in a couple of weeks.'

'In your experience, is there evidence that these exercises improve the amount of sensation during penetrative sex?'

'Yes, these exercises are good for the health of the bladder, to avoid rectal prolapse, they prevent incontinence when women get older and, yes, it definitely improves the sex life too.'

The nerve endings are in the muscles, you see.

'I'll work hard at these exercises.'

'But no breaking the flow of urine on the loo. We don't recommend that.'

'My GP told me that that's how you find out if your PC (pubococcygeus) muscle is strong or not.'

I saw Clare shudder slightly. 'No, there is a little more to it than that.'

'What about all the toys that are available out there to help?'

'We don't recommend the beads of various kinds because they encourage women to lift up rather than bringing the muscles forward toward the pelvic bone.'

She pulls a model out of a drawer that shows the muscles in two layers. 'You want this band of muscle to pull up and forwards.'

'Up and forward? OK. I've also seen, online, women discussing that if you are doing lots of pelvic floor exercises then it's good to squat too. They recommend peeing in the shower as it makes women squat right down fully the way a child does and this apparently stretches the muscles the other way.'

'We also recommend Pilates as a general training for all the core muscles of that part of the body. It all helps. It changed the shape of the bottom half of my boss's body, she is fond of saying. So many women worry about having saggy tummies but it's not as if we can't do anything about these muscles.'

'I'll start with my *pube rectalis* then.' It would be wrong not to.

• • •

I have been open with my friends on Facebook about the fact that I'm working on a book about sexuality. So I receive all kinds of weird invitations.

Take this one. 'Isabel, would you like to join me on a three-day training with the incredible Dossie Easton, author of *The Ethical Slut*, and general matriarch of the modern tantric/BDSM[25] hybrid movement. Almost 70 and still tying up, flogging and circular breathing with the best?'

Me: 'Why do we need to tie up and flog people that we love?'

'It's about creating polarity, like the electrical charge on a battery. Lightning moves between polarites. We don't do anything we don't want to do with people we love. This is about learning how to create an intense energetic exchange between people and building energetic capacity.'

I'm unusually silent. He goes on,

'I've done a fair bit of yoga, meditation and solo spiritual practice in my life, and polarity work (tantric BDSM, Taoist sexuality practice) is by far the most powerful I've ever experienced. Tying up and flogging is one of a thousand ways we create a charge. The other part to it is to learn the dance of hormones and neuro-transmitters. If played just right the crescendo of dopamine and oxytocin is exquisite, transcendental and, coincidentally, very similar in brain wave and endocrine profile to what happens when experienced meditators report "enlightenment" experiences.'

Maybe I'm deeply dull. I said, 'No, thank you.' I saw the lash marks on this man's back after the workshop. But you can find Dossie if this sounds like an area you'd like to explore.[26]

There seem to be organizations teaching sexuality of one kind or another popping up like mushrooms. One night I get invited to an event where I sit and get told about 11 different types of orgasm – ten of which I haven't had. Let me run this information by you and I hope your score is higher than mine.

Firstly, there is the famous 'clitoral' orgasm. Even these aren't easy for many women but most sexuality schools will teach that this is definitely not what it's all about. They are often quick and not satisfying we get told. I wonder at these evenings how many women sit feeling guilty. Sheesh. Then I sit listening again to hear that vaginal orgasms may be a little better but not if they are created by 'friction'. But I've heard this from more than one school (I'm not allowed to name names here, sadly, as I know this is very interesting). 'Friction-based vaginal orgasms' are also not encouraged as they are over too quickly and don't help us reach our orgasmic potential. And of course others encourage us not to think about our orgasmic potential at all and just – once again – to think about sensation.

My dentist (she of the worshipped yoni) went to an evening with tantric teacher Saby Harmony in London in a basement at Neal's Yard. Most Londoners think this is just a place for good organic food and herbs but you just never know who is hiring out the basement. She tells me that she went to a night there that started with people choosing partners, enjoying extensive eye contact, establishing boundaries and expressing where they were happy to be touched. This she confides over a coffee when she's finished drilling my teeth one week. She told her partner he could touch her anywhere he wanted as long as it was external. Her exercise was just to give him feedback. If I'd had the courage I wish I'd spent evenings like this when I was 19. It would have changed my life. As it is I wouldn't have the courage to do this even now. Anyway – to speed up the story the massage was about two hours (apparently they took a long time to get to the intimate bits) but it did end up including extensive genital pleasure while she simply gave him feedback. She was completely safe of course because she was in a room with a facilitator to instruct, observe and make sure that established boundaries were maintained. And there is a group of other people doing the same. Does everyone else know that these kind of events are happening in London?

But back to the different types of orgasm that I haven't had.

There is the 'squirting orgasm' – that's the one with female ejaculation. Some women describe this as a different type of orgasm. But maybe we shouldn't count this one as, strictly speaking, it's just an orgasm where a woman 'ejaculates' at the same time. This is said to be very good for women's health and is all the rage in Germany – as you'll remember.

Then there is the curious 'G-spot orgasm'. Controversy be gone. One tantra school I visited was very sure – we have one, they say. It feels like a walnut and it's two inches inside women on the front wall. You can find it as the skin has a different texture from the skin around it. I desperately want to argue and say, 'But surely all women's bodies are different?' But when you attend tantric events that allow you to keep your clothes on it's really best to limit the questions to nine or ten as the organizers do have a certain amount of material to get through.

Did you ever see a film called *Deep Throat*? I didn't – I was probably watching something far more innocent when other more liberated people were watching this. Apparently it features the 'mouth or throat orgasm'. I'm reliably informed that if women can learn to overcome the gagging reflex and can insert the 'cock' (no fancy yoni/lingam language at the evening I went to when they talked about this one) far enough down her throat, this will make a woman orgasm in her throat. Any takers?

Some women have more luck. I recently spoke to a girlfriend who tells me that she has spontaneous orgasms during meditation. During meditation?! I spent over ten days doing Vipassana meditation for ten hours a day with Goenka's teaching and all I got for it was pain. Lots and lots of pain. And some women are having spontaneous orgasms during meditation? Have I been doing the wrong courses? If you are a course that teaches how to achieve this, please write to me and I'll do another book and tell you all how I learnt.

The anal orgasm – easier for some women than others apparently. I've heard that it only leads to orgasm if your kundalini is opened. And how do you open your kundalini? I've no idea.

I asked a friend who is a yoga teacher.

'Is your kundalini open?'

'Open is one term. Awakened is another. "Kunda Lini" means the coiled serpent.'

'OK, so is your serpent uncoiled?'

'We've all had these experiences.'

'No. I'm quite sure my serpent is coiled. So is yours uncoiled?'

'It's a higher state of consciousness. I've read yogic texts ...' (Hasn't everyone? No?) She goes on.

'... that describe experiences you have as the serpent awakens and spirals up the Sushumna ...'

'My what?'

'The central energy motorway of the body that criss-crosses at the chakras. You know that Rod of Asclepius that doctors have?'

'No.'

'A snake wrapped around a central staff?'

'No.'

She looks at me surprised.

'But anyway,' I ask, 'is your kundalini open or awakened or what?'

'Yes. Why are you asking?'

'I heard that people can only have anal orgasms if their kundalini are open.'

'I think that's bollocks.'

I think I'll leave that conversation there and not cross-examine her any further about the connection between higher states of consciousness and anal penetration.

'So, er, seen any good films recently?'

So back to the 11 different forms of orgasm. An all-women's event spoke about a 'Valley Orgasm'. To learn what a Valley orgasm is they recommended reading *Tantric Orgasm for Women*. So if any of you want to understand this one I'll put this book in the appendix with the other books. There is certainly a lot of pleasure available to us isn't there?

There is also the 'A-spot orgasm'. I'm way behind. I'm still looking for the G-spot. Apparently the A-spot is 3–4 inches deep on the front wall of the vagina. And there is the 'Cervix' or 'Womb' orgasm. This is apparently achieved by hitting the back of the vagina on the cervix. At an introduction evening for a tantra course that I went to in Brighton (this one was mixed) I saw a woman do a *When Harry met Sally* demo of her experience during a Cervical orgasm and it certainly didn't resemble anything I've ever experienced.

Later a friend reminds me, after reading this, that she once had a 'Breast Orgasm'. Apparently women can learn to orgasm just having our breasts rubbed? Men, don't you want to learn this? And then one of my German friends who is training as a sexual body worker with Mike Lousada (no relation) tells me she knows how to have what she called a 'Mental Orgasm' just by thinking and exercising her pelvic floor muscles. Apparently she imagines that the Hindu god, Shiva, is making love to her. Sheesh, my dreams are dull.

And not only my dreams. Sometimes exploring all this makes me think that I'm just wildly normal. Thinking that maybe we had got a bit diverted by the more esoteric pathways, T and I decided to visit the London 'Sexpo' exhibition at Olympia. 'Sexpo' is a health, sexuality and lifestyle exhibition and is 'the world's longest running adult exhibition and is designed to provide a fun, vibrant and safe environment for open-minded adults.' But this is certainly the other extreme. It was mainly stalls selling sex toys and dressing-up clothes of all kinds. Women made of rubber lay on the floor in interesting positions.

'I've never seen so many dildos in one building,' T said, as we wandered down exhibition-style rows of stalls seemingly with every sex shop in Europe represented. There were dressing-up clothes of all kinds and for all sexes, scantily-clothed women dancing around poles, and scantily-clothed men strutting on stage.

'Did you say you'd like to get a dog?' T asked randomly. But then I looked around and there was a man in a full bodysuit dressed as a dog. On his hands and knees crawling about with groups of other human dogs all doing 'Puppy play'.

'They're human pups,' said a woman cheerfully, seeing my confused face. 'Would you like to pat one?' A man knelt before me in a 'sit up and beg' position, panting with his tongue out. 'Er – good dog,' I patted him as seemed to be required. T laughed at seeing me utterly confused and went to get tea.

'I think I'm in the wrong place again,' I sighed. 'Look, they even have single-use plastic cups. I can't handle this.' 'What – the human dogs?'

I can't handle the human dogs, the plastic cups or the plastic lids. Our poor oceans. 'I really don't need a lid, thanks. I'm going to drink this tea right now,' I barked, rather grumpily, at the poor girl serving tea.

'And breathe out.' T smiled at me getting vexed.

'Is there anything to do here apart from ogle half-dressed flesh or buy weird stuff for fetishes we don't have?' I grumbled.

'There are some interesting talks. Here's one called "To Cum or Not to Cum, Is That a Question?" For men? Well, that's different.'

'It's about the male not ejaculating? OK, let's go and hear what this Drew Lawson has to say'.[27]

So we went and sat among a small audience that contained some very interestingly-dressed people and listened to the debate about whether the ancient Asian idea that it's not good for a man to ejaculate too often is true or not.

A lot of the men in the audience were from the 'I want to ejaculate as often as I possibly can' school of action. Their reasons included: it feels good, helps me relax, helps me sleep, I feel deeply connected to everything, my mind stops thinking about my job and for a few seconds I become bliss and I feel less tense and more mellow after I ejaculate. Also a woman added that she enjoys making her man ejaculate.

Drew Lawson (tall, good-looking, well-spoken and well-dressed) was explaining the alternative perspective while I scribbled notes rapidly. The Indian Vedic teachings suggest that ejaculation drains our 'Ojas'. Apparently this is some form of our 'vital essence' which they say is difficult or impossible to replace – our life energy if you like. As sperm does contain life energy I suppose this makes sense.

The average man (if there is such a man?) lasts under ten minutes during sexual intercourse'. The 'average woman' takes more than 30 minutes of sexual intimacy and physical connection to 'start to move into orgasmic states'. Are you finding this very reassuring, women? I was. I wish I could have given this specific piece of information to a 25-year-old version of me. Once a woman is in an orgasmic state this can continue for hours. This, Drew said, very reasonably, may be 'reason enough' for men to learn how to have conscious choice over their ejaculatory response.

Then there is the question of hormones. Scientific studies in animals suggest that ejaculation spikes dopamine, oxytocin and prolactin levels in the body, which then can drop to low levels and take nearly three weeks to return to a normal level. Men who practice non-ejaculation say that after three weeks their bodies feel happier, healthier and that they have more energy and have been able to be more focused on their lovers.

Also, they are still having orgasms (this much I remembered). Practitioners suggest that by not ejaculating they can build a different and deeper orgasmic sensation in their bodies, which have been described, variously, as heart orgasms, spine orgasms, full-body orgasms and pineal orgasms. Oh goodness – yet more names for different types of orgasms. Apparently people report orgasmic sensations in different locations in the body – sometimes called the 'chakra' locations, sometimes called 'energy centres' in yoga and the location of nerve plexuses in anatomy and physiology.

A couple of men asked if he was talking bullshit. (There is a lot of straight talking at the Sexpo exhibition.) So Drew said,

'In my personal experience, when I have more than about 15 days of non-ejaculation in my body, I feel more alive, more vital, focused, connected, energized and present.' He chose his words carefully to describe the sensation.

'How does this impact on your sex with your women if you don't cum?' asked a man sceptically and with a strange degree of antagonism.

'I feel more able to meet her and be in deep intimacy with her. I feel more as if I'm serving and giving her my energy rather than taking or using her to scratch an itch.'

'I like that description of bad sex ...' said a shapely woman in the back row. 'It's honestly felt like that sometimes – as though I'm being used to scratch an itch.' She made a fast and vigorous scratching movement with her hand. We laughed and sighed.

'It makes sex much more intimate,' said another woman. 'Yes, we felt that when my lover and I did this for a month.' Drew was just sharing information. 'After more than 50 or 60 days I feel as if my body is humming with vitality and energy.'

I just went on making notes, interested to see how T would respond. I half expected him to say, 'No way!' But as ever he's full of surprises.

'I want to try this,' he said, when the talk had ended. 'I think it will be interesting.'

'You do?'

'It'll be interesting for me to see how long I can go without ejaculating.'

'Will this mean less sex or more sex?'

'I'm just going to ask him some more questions.' He returned smiling.

'Neither. It doesn't mean having sex more or less often, it just means that I don't ejaculate and also, if I masturbate, I don't ejaculate. I thought I'd experiment.'

Obviously Drew doesn't own this practice. No one owns this any more than the OM lot own clitoral stroking – they are both ancient tantric exercises. Just teachers of sexuality like Drew recommend trying them.

So T accepted the challenge and made it past 20 days and I can fill you in a bit on the exercise. Part of the time he was travelling and we weren't together. I'm not sure whether this made it harder or easier for him but I can report the following: on day nine he sent me a text, 'I think this is already a record for me since puberty.'

'You mean if you weren't doing this you'd be masturbating to ejaculation every day when we're not together?'

'Yes. Blokes do that, you know. It feels good and it helps me sleep. Why wouldn't I?'

'I don't know. It's just that, er, most women I know don't do it every day. You think most blokes do?'

'Yes.'

It's not a question we ever ask really, is it?

On other days he'd just text me, 'Day 12' or 'Day 14', as if he was notching up some huge accomplishment. 'Many men don't make it to this many days,' he said proudly.

'Notice anything?' I asked on Day 16. 'I have a lot more time on my hands. So to speak. An extra 10–20 minutes a day and when I say "I'm going to my room to read a book," I'm actually reading a book.'

On the days when we did see each other during this time I really enjoyed our lovemaking. Everything seems to teach slowing down. Be more mindful. Breathe together more. Enjoying subtlety with him focusing on not ejaculating helped this process. It made it more like coasting and less like driving. We had already removed the goal for me and so removing the goal for him too brought us into greater balance. Like a dance that was more in time. It didn't feel as though he was dancing to one drum and I was dancing to another. Maybe it made him better able to 'listen' to my body rather than being overtaken. And of course it meant we could enjoy everything for longer.

On day 18 he said, 'I feel as if I have more energy and more sexual energy but I don't know whether I'm imagining it or not.'

'Are you still sleeping OK?'

'Yes. It's good to know I can just get into bed and fall asleep with er ... no extra effort.'

On day 25, which was the target he had set himself, I had a boyfriend who was very keen to see me. [T: 'You need to write "very" in caps there, Isabel.' I: 'It's OK, they get it.']

He's enjoying this year of exploration of all kinds. It's not always easy for either of us: For him, being anonymous; for me, half wanting to tell you all about him but not being able to because he's a real person. It's not easy this journey for either of us – but it has good moments. Velvet moments. Sometimes we may both feel like jumping ship. But neither of us is sorry to be on this journey. If this whole project was a bookable cruise – would you want a ticket?

What's Love Got to Do with It?

The following morning Alexey rings. He asks how I'm getting on with everything.

I tell him about all the strange evenings I've been hearing about and attending. I tell him about the Sexpo exhibition. About the human dogs. There's a pause down the line.

'Would you like to meet for a coffee?'

'Yes – I would.'

I tell him all my adventures.

'These talks, these experiences, seminar introduction nights, exhibitions ... Has anyone mentioned love at all?'

I think about it. 'Well, er, no. Not specifically.'

'Very few teachers seem to mention it. I feel as if I've invented it.'

I laugh. I'm assuming, in this book, that we are on this journey because there is, or may at some point in the future be, someone that we feel love for ... but of course then we have to define what we mean by love. Always a tricky one ...

So, with the help of coffee, we consider this topic.

Alexey is in a mild state of shock at my stories.

'How can any of the organizations or seminars or anyone that teaches sexuality do a whole evening on sex and not mention love? Sex just for pleasure is meaningless. That's why there are so many couples watching TV.'

'Surely people are watching TV because they are not having any pleasure?'

'Even if they're having pleasure, it has to be about love. The deepest connection is potentially to yourself, your partner and your life. This connection in lovemaking has the power to impact your life in a very deep way. No matter how good a blow job is, it just doesn't have that impact.'

'OK, Alexey – but what's love anyway?' Always an

interesting question I think.

'Love is energy.'

'You said last time that sex is energy.'

'It's all energy isn't it?'

'Yes.'

'But how can a woman express love through penetrative sex with, for example, a husband who has annoyed her that day and she's feeling very little sensation?'

'That's a bit like when someone asked Mooji, "How do I learn to trust again? I'm heart-broken." And he says, "That's not your heart, that's just stuff in your head that can't trust. That's not the real heart."'

'I can see that to an extent. We all listen to our thoughts too much and it is possible to let things go.'

'In sex we are so obsessed with consuming. Taking turns and doing jobs for each other doesn't count. That's like saying, "I'll be your toy if you'll be my toy later. You focus on your consumerism and I'll focus on mine." But your energy is what comes from you; it's not about what you receive. What makes you alive, what makes you feel is what comes out of you.'

'St Francis said that.'

'What?'

'Not in a sexual context. Evidently. Sorry ... you were saying?'

'Love in sex is enjoying someone and making someone feel good, wanting to give something to someone. If we are not strangers just working each other there is an energy that comes from our bodies – energy that wants the other to be well. We give energy that is a caring gift. Love in sex is being able to give the energy of your heart with your body – you breathe life into a person and you leave something good with them. They come charged with your love. And then there is the enjoying the aesthetic in sex. Loving can also mean honouring someone very much – touching a body with respect. You have been allowed to touch and so it's about enjoying all the senses.'

'You make it sound very beautiful, Alexey.'

'This is what I teach.'

'How strange that you should have to teach this.'

'I teach these two aspects. In the moment of sex itself you need to know how to evoke your own energies and to really appreciate the other person rather than just worrying about making it work.'

'But say someone has a partner and the main energy that he or she is carrying around is anger, anxiety, sadness, depression, fear, neediness, resentment, pain or any combination of those – then what that person has to share is that troubled energy because that is the main energy that is dominating their mind, body and spirit.'

'It's irrelevant.'

'Why?'

'Because I'm talking about what we can express. Love is your energy.'

'And that can't be abused? Taken advantage of?'

'Yes, but I'm assuming a certain amount of common sense. After all we choose who we give our love to. I'm assuming we're talking about a situation where both partners are choosing to be in the same bed.'

'OK. That is where I started actually. A couple that just want their sex to be as good as it can be.'

'The return each partner gets is not what they are given but what they give. The return you get is in the moment of giving. When people talk about sex it's only relatively recently that the first thing that comes to mind is all the weirdness associated with it. The first context that you associate it with is love.'

'I think maybe that love used to be the first thing that people associated with sex. Of course in traditional religions the ideal is that you only get to enjoy this with someone when you love them so much you want to spend your whole life with them.'

'It has all got a bit dark hasn't it? And it is possible to have sex without love. You can do it in an S&M way and be beating each other and you may get something enjoyable out of it. But personally I don't believe that real happiness can be found there.'

'No? Wouldn't those who enjoy those expressions of their sexuality say that we have limited understanding of love expressed in that way?'

'I think it's unstable.'

'It's very different from what you teach.'

'Love is the core of sex. I'm not saying that I only teach love, but love is the core of the energy and if it's absent it's never going to be complete. A lot of things we feel, physically, hinge on that. The happiness that you feel from sex comes from that.'

'So, maybe I just don't love my partner enough? Maybe

many of us don't really know how to love our partners enough? How do you "love" all the people that come to you? You don't love all your clients.'

'I love them in the sacred space that is created there; I give love with energy and touch. In that space my love is my energy. Out of that space they are just people again but that loving energy stays with them. I don't need to like them. People don't need to like their partners in order to love them with a loving sexual energy.'

I can hear some of you readers checking out in that last paragraph. You may be thinking, 'What is this guy on about?' Is it easier to love relative strangers for a while than to love the man who hasn't taken the rubbish out or the woman who has just maxed out the joint credit card? Sorry about the stereotypes there.

'It's irrelevant.'

'Is it? I must be missing something. Please can you go back to your definition of love? You are saying, "Love is the key ingredient in sexuality." OK, so how are you defining "love" in this context?'

He paused and then reached over and touched my arm.

'If I put my hand on you I want you to feel that I want you to feel good. I want your body, right now, in that place where I'm touching you to feel happy, to feel cared for. I don't want to just touch your body in a way that will press buttons so that you get a desire in your genitals. At this place in your body where I'm touching you I want you to feel that the sun has come or the rain has come. There is something that brings you alive from this contact with me. I want you to experience that when I take my hand away there will be something that stays there. I really do feel, in my heart, that I want to give something to you that will stay with you. I want you to be well and I want you to be happy afterwards. In this moment I am the only person who can make you feel loved. Right now I am the only source of that unique kind of love that humans have between each other. There may be someone else in your life but right now there is only me.'

'Simple human warmth?'

'In a way. I want, through this touching, with all the sensations and pleasure, to share the warmth of my soul. I also want to love the beauty of you. I want to touch you and I want to feel how beautiful this is. How it feels, the curves of it. I'm touching something beautiful and I'm grateful for this opportunity. I just want to explore it and savour every second. I want to deepen more into that. And that makes you feel appreciated and loved. So ... that's the difference compared to someone thinking that maybe if they touch her there, really well, then she'll get a spark up and then eventually maybe she'll have an orgasm.'

'Sex can be exhausting when it becomes about that.'

'Exactly. That sex is exhausting with an orgasm and this sex is recharging without one. If I touch you well for even five minutes, you'll feel better than after orgasm-chasing sex. Sometimes you even lose energy and so does the man. All these techniques they speak of, they just fall off. But with love – beauty will awaken inside you, and with that more sensitivity. The giver and the receiver – they don't exist anymore.'

'Your words are like poetry, Alexey. But I'm still left asking how is it possible for any woman to give this kind of love to a man who is a criminal, a compulsive addict or even, as I said, a husband who they are usually fond of but who will not take the rubbish out?'

'I'd say the third of the three is the bigger problem. I mean we mess up in a million ways but we can still go into that energy – she can still be a woman that can enjoy bringing something good to him to counteract the bad. And the chances are that those first two men, even though they have failed, will give her some love too. But the one who hasn't taken the rubbish out is going to get her really annoyed – at the time itself, so she may be feeling really negative energy in her body, because it feels as though he isn't respecting her. So that will take her more effort, in that moment, to overcome.'

'Well, and the partners of the other two, surely as well? What about a man who is emotionally abusive? And the men too – as I said earlier. It's hard to love a woman who may, for example, have compulsively lied to you. Or who mocks you – or who sometimes just isn't kind.'

'That's why the concept of sacred space exists. When you go into the sacred sexual space it's all about the energy field in that moment. All the other stuff has to be left outside.'

'I'm pleased that I know someone like you exists.'

'Thank you. Where did that come from?'

'I'm so pleased that someone uses words like those or understands these things. I remember feeling, in several relationships where the sex wasn't like this, that a man must exist who would be interested in kissing me and be glad to do so. Not because I'm special but because everyone is special. To be with any other human being is an honour, as you say. I remember thinking to myself that love is about energy because a man lay beside me once and shook, but there is so much that tells us that sex is – well, what do you call it?'

'Friction and novelty techniques.'

'You are funny.'

'I've not heard anyone put this into words. It's consoling listening to you. Even the concept of the sacred space, of making love with someone in this way is beautiful.'

'You've read about it though?'

'I've read the poetry of Rumi. But when most people talk about "creating a sacred space" they are usually talking about putting down some red cushions and lighting candles.'

'That makes me laugh.'

'But to be fair you mean that too. Create a beautiful environment and then make love but you don't really even need a beautiful environment, you can make love beautifully even in a messy room.'

'So everything else has to be left outside.'

'Yes.'

'Don't miss the miracle of being alive and having a body and senses. You can give someone happiness and joy just by touching them.'

'Yes. No matter how good the "pleasure" factor, if you feel miserable the following day, it's not good sex. And if it gives you lasting happiness and joy that IS good sex. That's just my stance.'

I love these words. They make sense to me.

Winter by the Fire

Take a Deep Breath

S o the last of the leaves are falling from the trees outside today. Instead of sitting at my desk I'm sitting on the sofa with a hot water bottle and a blanket.

I know that there are several pieces missing on my quest. The most important, I feel instinctively, is the breath. The whole subject of breathing and the breath is key to vitality and to sexuality. I don't know this because I've experienced it fully. I know it because, well, I feel it. I'm convinced that the fact that we hold our breath and don't breathe correctly is one of the key causes for much of our 'dis-ease'.

It's not just during sex – most of us don't breathe correctly all the time. I remember years ago I was reading my old friend do-you-want-to-murder-him-Anthony-Robbins on the subject of excellence. He claims, quite logically, that before we can be excellent at anything we need energy, and in order to have energy he doesn't suggest buying a product or taking one of his seminars. He talks about breathing. He writes about the lymph system and its importance to the body. Then he points out that although the blood has a heart to pump it around the body, lymphatic fluid (which is vital for the immune system) does not. What is vital in moving the lymph around the body? Deep breathing. What oxygenates the blood and keeps us healthy? Deep breathing. What gives life and vitality to every cell in the body? Oxygen through ... deep breathing. He says, 'Look carefully at any "health programme" that doesn't first and foremost teach you how to fully cleanse your body through effective breathing.' He writes that if you get nothing else from his writing apart from an understanding of the importance of correct breathing, you could dramatically increase the level of your body's health. And this is what he recommends in his book, *Unlimited Power*. He asks that, three times a day, you breathe in to a count of one then hold for a count of four and breathe out to a count of two. Build up your breathing daily at that ratio until you can, comfortably and without straining, lead up to breathing in for a count of seven, holding your breath for a count of 28 and breathing out for a count of 14. He says that this creates a vacuum that sucks lymph through the bloodstream and multiplies the pace at which the body eliminates toxins. Now, is that true? I have no idea. But I do know how it makes me feel when I do this kind of breathing, which is energized.

And what has this got to do with sex, you ask? Bear with me. I'm just talking about breathing a bit.

There was an experience I had with 're-birthing'. This is the discipline which, according to The British Rebirth Society, 'brings into awareness not only our unconsciously held beliefs and emotions' but also the relationships we have with 'our bodies, ourselves and our world'. When we breathe with this awareness, they say we make it possible to 'resolve, integrate and heal previously unresolved issues within ourselves'. And how do they do this? In the presence of an experienced breath worker, you breathe a full and relaxed breath with no pause between the in-breath and out-breath. When you do this for between 30 and 50 minutes (don't try it at home alone) you take in more oxygen than you usually would, which increases the levels of CO_2 in the brain. This leads you into a semi-trance-like state in which all kinds of weird things happen. Both mental and even physical memories emerge. For example, you may feel a pain from an injury that you believe was healed long ago. Or you may find yourself sobbing about some loss that you thought forgotten. It's weird. And my point is? The breath is powerful and changes our state.

If you just imagine, vividly, right this minute that someone is about to give you an injection in your arm. Put your right arm out and look the other way. If you have imagined it well you may find that you are holding your breath. We do this if some part of us doesn't want to feel a sensation. And we get into bad habits.

Here is another way to experiment with how breath influences you. A breath-work teacher and Kundalini practitioner, Susan P. Boles in Canada, studied breath-work after a severe spinal injury. She writes of a method where she was taught by breathing in to four slow counts. She says, 'Feel the breath expand your ribcage ... you are aiming to fill your whole chest cavity with air. At the end of the fourth, when you think you can't take any more air in, take a sip more.' Then you hold for a count of four before exhaling over a count of four. She says that when you think all the air is gone then breathe out some more, assuring us that there is more that can be breathed out even when we think our lungs are empty.

She writes, 'You may experience burning in your lungs doing this. But soon, your breathing comes deep and sure. The count of four expands to a count of five or six.' Then she invites us to concentrate on the emptiness between breathing in and breathing out ... that period of stillness.

Then she talks about the practice of 'breathing in from different parts of the body' that I hear about from many sources. Then I read the instruction to breathe through my genitals. I sigh. What? 'Breathe in through my genitals?' I ask with my literal brain being a little dominant. 'Er?' But Susan writes that she discovered various weird and woo woo things were possible just practising breathing. She says, 'Once my lungs were used to doing this, I started to visualize breathing in from different parts of my body. No one taught me this, it just started to happen when I meditated.'

She would imagine opening up the top of her head or her 'crown chakra' and breathing in through there on the in-breath, on the pause she would imagine the energy flowing around her heart chakra and then on the out-breath push the breath through the rest of her body and out through her feet. No one suggests that this is possible literally but there is something about imagining breathing into those places that seems to energize them in a way that we don't fully understand.

Continuing her experiments, she imagines breathing in through her feet, holding it around her heart and breathing out 'through her head'.

She says, 'It was dizzying at first but energy fills me when I do this; that's incredible.'

Then there is the famous 'Breath of Fire' technique. Kundalini yoga teacher Anne Novak claims that just practising this technique for five minutes a day 'will strengthen your heart, your lungs and your nervous system'. She says that purifying and oxygenating your blood in this way will give you tremendous energy and even says that if you do this practice it will deepen the way you breathe for the rest of the day which will give you a steady energy not dependent on 'pick-me-ups' like tea and coffee and that you'd 'be able to face life's challenges with grace and joy'.[28]

This is a pretty strong claim for a five-minute breathing technique. So here it is. Sit with a straight spine and place your hand on your diaphragm. Take a deep breath and then using your diaphragm and tummy muscles (very technical here) push all the breath out, with a sound. Then let the air enter in naturally. Then push it out again. Repeat this, initially at one breath a second and then raise it to two breaths a second. Your hand isn't resting there to do the pushing; it's just there so that you can feel your diaphragm going in. It's not so much breath – rather like a whoosh out and a gentle draw in. There is a very good demo of this on YouTube. You'll find it at 'Breath of Fire: Kundalini Yoga basics.'

Then there is 'alternative nostril breathing' where you breathe in through one nostril then block it and breathe out through the other; then in again through the one you've breathed out of. Then you block that and breathe out through the first. And so on. This one is a slower breath and is simply used to calm you down. It does calm you down.

Then there is the 'Ujjayi breath' in Hatha yoga (again you can look all these different breathing practices up on YouTube). This breathing practice actually means 'to be victorious'. Such are the claims made on your behalf if you are prepared to become a master of your breath.

And all this is possible even if you don't do yoga or don't want to do yoga. Even if you are bedridden. If you are alive, you can explore the breath.

Then, outside the field of yoga there is an amazing and comparatively little-known Russian breathing technique called 'The Buteyko Method'.[29] This completely natural breathing teaching reverses asthma and helps even children gain control over and eventually free themselves from their inhalers. They use fun breathing games that include holding your breath and learning how to redress the symptoms that lead to asthma attacks. The Buteyko Method is also used to treat high blood pressure and irritable bowel syndrome. You don't even have to own a yoga mat to learn about this.

The reason I'm telling you all this is that I want to consider the importance of the breath to sensation. I don't think any of us have any clue how important it is to breathe well unless we are breath-workers. I don't think we realize how much we hold our breath or the effect of shallow breathing on our health. I don't think we realize the spiritual significance of breathing. I have certainly never heard a sermon on it in any church.

The Holy Spirit is mostly linked to the notion of breath and life. A priest friend reminds me that the word 'spirit' etymologically means 'breath'. This is how we get the word 'respiration'. Then, in ancient Greek you have 'pneuma' meaning both 'life force' (which has given us 'pneumonia', a disease of the lungs) and 'pneumatic' meaning containing and operated by air. That's us of course – we are beings containing and operated by air. And in ancient Hebrew and Semitic languages, 'Ruach' means 'wind' or 'life-giving breath' – but not just any old 'life'. It means what we would call 'spiritual life'. So there is a very close connection between what we call the breath and what we might call 'Life', 'The Source', 'The Holy Spirit' or, even, 'God'.

And of course our breath is our surest friend. There are few things of which we can be sure. One is that we will die and another is that until that time we have breath and that this breath gives us not only our life, but the quality of our life depending on the quality of the breath.

I've a friend who is an engineer and for his PhD he designed breathing machines for those whose lungs have been ruined by emphysema. I was reading his dissertation, understanding nothing of the engineering but there was something about the dry language that made it all the more horrific. He described the simple fact that patients who depend on machines for breath would rather be dead but they don't have the courage to switch off the machines and suffocate. These patients can't inhale any more. So the machines have to force the air in, which makes them want to gag at every in-breath. Then the out-breath comes naturally as the machine pauses and the lungs simply release. But then the machine forces air in again. And so on. I read my way through descriptions of why each of the current machines is ghastly and that there is really no less agonizing solution. My job, in theory, was simply to copyedit. But sadly my imagination meant that I visualized the patients.

'Did you meet these people?' I asked.

'Yes,' he said. 'It wasn't pretty.'

The clergyman who answered my questions about the breath sits regularly and holds people's hands as they die 'drowning in the tar inside their own lungs'. I will not write my feelings about the tobacco industry.

But for the rest of us, who can still breathe without the help of a machine, have you ever explored the breath? How it relates to energy and sex?

I have a feeling that my lack of understanding about the breath has influenced my sexual experience all my life. And T's too for that matter. T's 25-day challenge proved to be a perfect time to explore the influence of the breath on the body. I remember hearing a story once about a sex and relationship coach who had more clients than he had time for. He would meet each of them once and tell them, before they made love, to experiment with breathing together for 30 minutes. Apparently very few of them ever returned. Why? Well, possibly because they found this advice annoying or possibly because they tried it.

The reason it works is that if you and your partner are on what some people might call different frequencies then it helps you to tune in with each other. This beautiful exercise needs to be done facing each other.

Traditionally the woman leads the rhythm of the breathing

and the man follows her. It's difficult at first and you feel as if you are going to hyperventilate, you've forgotten how to breathe, you're too hot or your hands go buzzy or all kinds of weird things happen. But just keep breathing. Eventually you'll calm down and feel as if a gentle stream of energy is running between you. It is.

This is the energy that Alexey speaks about and of which we may not always be aware. Anyone who has studied physics will tell us that we are made up of a mixture of space, water and energy. If you study Vipassana or any form of yoga you may even have experienced a sensation as if you are a being made purely of energy, and that the muscles and bones don't seem to belong to that which is you. It may seem a weird way to begin to come together with someone in an act that is of the body, but I'm not suggesting that you do this every night. You need to experience yourselves as energetic bodies and have even a glimpse of how your energies come together, meld and influence each other. This is why you need half an hour.

It's a little bit special. I don't want to tell you too much about my experience this time. I want you to go away and experience it for yourself.

And to explore energetic exchange and the breath you don't even need a sexual partner. The monks and nuns of Thích Nhat Hanh's community in southwest France have a very special way of hugging, they call it 'hugging meditation'. In the description on their website they write that,

'When we hug our hearts connect and we know that we are not separate beings.'

But to be reminded of this they have a very special way of hugging that involves a lot of deep breathing. They meet and then, instead of doing a quick polite hug with no body contact, they first pause. Then they stand and take three deep breaths to make sure that they are fully present. Then they open their arms and give 'full body' hugs, which they maintain for a further three deep breaths. During the first inhalation and exhalation they focus on being grateful for being present in that very moment and being happy to be there. (We can assume you wouldn't be hugging if you weren't happy to do so.) On the second inhalation and exhalation they become fully aware of the presence of the other and are happy that the other is there. On the third breath in and out they focus on gratitude for being together in the present moment, on this earth. They focus on deep gratitude and happiness for this togetherness. Then they bow to each other. They say, 'We hug in such a way that the other person becomes real and alive to us.' These people are celibate monks and nuns.

It's a pretty good example for those of us that are about to have sex, wouldn't you say? Surely we could, sometimes, potentially at least, be honouring each other at least as much as if we are going to get naked with and touch our bits together? Or if we are in a couple where we're considering making love in order to create new life, could this be something sacred? Be 'dirty' some nights – whatever that means to you, if you like it like that, and 'sacred' on others? Sometimes? Maybe? Just saying.

But back to breathing before sex. So, following deeper breathing, everything slows down naturally. T and I moved to making love and T slowed down his breathing. That was it. Result? A totally different form of sexual experience. Now if you've already been having the kind of sex where you both breathe very slowly and the man doesn't ejaculate, this may not be news to you. But for us it was just one more area that we hadn't explored before. The other piece of information that I had to play with, which I learnt at Hilly Spenceley's workshops, is that the man is supposed to follow the breathing of the woman. His physical movements coincide with my breath so when we arrive (finally) at penetration I can have him move just as slowly or as quickly as I like. I have to slow him down at times and become good at that. Or keep completely still if I like.

Now don't misunderstand me. I'm not saying that I always want control over my partner's breathing and movement in bed. But it is one more amazing area to experiment with. I hope T won't mind me telling you, because he is anonymous after all, that when his self-imposed 25-day challenge was over and we continued to explore this without the prohibition on ejaculation he experienced a 'totally new kind of orgasm'. One in which he was able to use the breath to slowly draw the sensation up from his genitals and through his body rather than having a genitally-centred orgasm.

I'm not yet at a place where I can pull sensation through my body using the breath. But I can use it for focus on sensation in different areas, and I do notice that if you put your mental focus on an area of your body and then you breathe in and think of bringing your energy to that area, for some reason you do feel more sensation in that area. Just don't ask me why or how this works, OK?

I wanted to check that my intuition about the breath was accurate even though no one seemed to be talking about it. So I phoned Sue Newsome of Shakti Tantra who had taken the couple's workshop that T and I had so much enjoyed. I simply said, 'Can you talk to me about the breath a bit, Sue?' 'Breathing is absolutely fundamental to our enjoyment of sexual pleasure,' she said. Ah. Very good.

'Say more please?'

'What can go wrong for some people in sex is that they are in their heads.' Again we hear this. No irrelevant thoughts, folks. No past, no future.

'By focusing on our breathing we are in our bodies rather than in our thoughts. We can use our breath to promote our arousal. The arousal can be harnessed using a combination of breath and muscle management.' (Those pelvic floor muscles again.) 'The breath is what takes the sensation through the whole body.'

'Imagine you can breathe in through your sex,' (for 'sex' here, read 'yoni', 'vulva' or 'perineum' as an option for men and women). 'Experiment with squeezing your pelvic floor muscles on the in-breath and relaxing them on the out-breath.'

Sheesh – we can have fun exploring the potential results of strong pelvic floor muscles and breathing deeply? You're really getting quite good value from this book. Explore though and find what works for you because advice differs. Alexey says, 'Don't focus on the breath, focus on the sensation, the breath will look after itself.' Some teachers advise, 'Don't worry about the breath, it will look after itself.' But almost everyone speaks of using the breath to draw sensation from your genitals up into the rest of the body.

From all the different types of orgasm that I haven't had – it's the one they call a 'Breath Orgasm' that I'd like to explore because the breath is our energy, our health, our sexuality, our spirituality. And there is a workshop that I could go to, and it doesn't involve taking my clothes off or touching strangers.

Just look at this. Go to your computer later and type these words in the search bar, 'How to have a breath and energy orgasm.' Or, if you're on an E-reader that can connect you just look here.[30] If you don't have a computer handy, this is a clip of a woman called Barbara Carrellas who, right there on camera, with no other person or object involved, breathes herself to this kind of orgasm in two minutes and ten seconds. So what on earth is going on here? How can she breathe herself to a kind of orgasm with no erotic stimulation of any kind?

I showed the clip to one of my German friends.

'Oh yes, this is an old tantric practice that we call "The Big Draw". I've done this in workshops in Germany.' Of course she has.

I find Barbara's website and scan the dates to find there is a one-day workshop that is four days after the wedding of a friend in New York. Just the excuse I'm looking for. The friend will give me air miles, I can stay for free and there is the wedding too. This makes it possible.

So, I shall go and learn how to breathe the body into some

kind of weird climax. And I'll teach you in case you are bored one night and want to explore how breathing may impact on whatever you do with the person that you love.

The Big Squeeze: Pelvic Floor II

You notice that we are running several themes at once here. Before we fly off to the US for the coldest winter on record we have an appointment with the NHS. I said I'd get back to you on the pelvic floor muscles exercise progress. If you are a female reader, are you doing them? Daily? Between my first and second meetings with Clare, I was disappointed with myself because, despite my best intentions, I didn't keep up the exercises with the five-times-a-day regularity that I had intended. I confessed this to her sorrowfully. Some days I had missed totally, intending to make up the pelvic floor squeezes on the following day. But, like any form of exercise, it doesn't work like that.

'Don't despair,' said Clare. 'Do you have a smart phone?'

'Yes.'

'There's an NHS app. It's a little controversial because, despite coming from the NHS, you have to pay for it.'

'How much?'

'£2.99.'

'Sold.'

We downloaded the app and Clare went through the exercises on it with me. It's called 'Squeezy'. Ha ha. And it has a selection of fast and slow squeezes along with the very important 'relax' section in which you need to make sure that you can also relax the muscles fully.

'We can set it for five times a day if you like?' said Clare cheerfully. 'It will send you reminders.'

And, oh my goodness, it does. It starts nagging at me at 9am and if I don't do it I get two messages saying 'Time for your 9am session.' Then it starts on me again at 11 and so on through the day. If I get behind it will say, 'You are three sessions overdue.' So now every time I get on a bus or a train or find myself waiting or sitting or even being driven in a car, I'll be sitting catching up on my daily Kegel muscles exercises. It's become like a good mixture of exercise and mediation as I concentrate on relaxing the breath and breathing slowly and steadily and pulling the pelvic floor muscles up and forward as much as I can. The first is slowly ten times, the second is fast ten times and the third is a more interesting 'half squeeze' that enables you to really feel what's going on.

If I'm still alive and have health problems in my 80s, then at least incontinence won't be one of them. Is it giving me more sensation during sex? Well apparently it's too early to say. I have to do these for at least eight weeks before I can expect to feel any change. But I'm becoming familiar with that part of my body. If this is 'The Ultimate Sex Secret Every Woman Should Know', I know it. Five times a day.

Sign up, girls. Get the app. Squeeze those sex muscles. And know how to relax and release them. For £2.99 you can look upon it as a contribution to the NHS. This, and links to other pelvic floor apps, are after the reading list at the end.

• • •

Those strange evenings in church halls and basements hearing a range of tantric and other sexuality teachers talking had raised questions that were still nagging at me. Does stimulation of the clitoris desensitize the vagina in any way or make other forms of orgasm apart from the clitoral orgasm less available? I think this question will be of considerable interest to a lot of us. It's difficult to answer the question definitively because, firstly, we know that the clitoris extends inside the vagina, so any study would have to be specific and limited to only the external clitoris. And then there is the vexed question of when is a clitoral orgasm a clitoral orgasm? Do we just mean that a non-clitoral orgasm is one in which the clitoris has not been touched? This makes no sense since the penis in penetration is obviously touching the clitoris – if not directly, then indirectly. Even the pressure of one body against another stimulates the clitoris through pressure against the hood. Gentle stroking with a very light touch has a different result on nerve endings from pushing a vibrator up against them. Bearing in mind the number of women who use vibrators – and mainly by stimulating the clitoris externally – this is an important question.

I write to Naomi Wolf (who spent years researching and writing a book called *Vagina*) and she writes back that she has never heard this and it makes no sense to her at all.

I wrote to Mike Lousada and he writes back with a fuller response,

'I'm not aware of any scientific evidence that points out that rubbing the clitoris desensitizes it (which doesn't mean that evidence doesn't exist, but I've not seen any and I've been doing this job a long time). I'd say that it's a matter of common sense.'

As a parallel, men who have circumcision have significantly less sensitivity around the head of the penis because it is unprotected, and constantly receives stimulation through friction. It follows therefore that overstimulating a clitoris may have the same impact. It would also depend on the type of stimulation. If it is gentle stroking, then my experience is that this opens up the nerve endings and creates greater sensitivity in a clitoris which may have become desensitized.

If the stimulation is intense and habitual, as in those women who only self-pleasure using a powerful vibrator, this can lead to desensitization of the area. Strong vibrators such as the Hitachi Wand should never be used directly on the skin. Women should place a wet flannel, folded over, between the vibrator and the genitals to ensure they don't overstimulate the sensitive area of the clitoris.

'Where I do sometimes recommend a vibrator is for women who have yet to experience orgasm and for whom regular touch does not seem to offer enough stimulation. In these cases I think of the vibrator like trainer-wheels on a bike – they give confidence when we're learning but should be disposed of as soon as possible.'

This is not the first time I've heard this. As that independent sex shop owner told T and me, women end up going back to sex shops to buy stronger vibrators. So if you have a clitoris and this is happening to you – stop. Put it away and stroke gently. Or go to an OM class.

Then I thought I'd ask Drew Lawson, who has studied with many of the different schools out there. He says,

'There seems to be a lot of conflict in the sex and intimacy world about "to clit or not to clit". There are some schools that focus entirely on clitoral stimulation, and others teach avoiding the clitoris altogether. However, as we know that the clitoral body is spread throughout the vagina, it's not just the small head under the clitoral hood. What seems to me to be more pertinent is which nerves are primarily activated by the different stimulations, and the effects those nerves have on the rest of the body and the endocrine system. The pudendal nerve inserts into the clitoris and when activated seems to create the pleasurable, spasmodic contractions that most of us associate with orgasm, along with the spike and crash in dopamine and oxytocin, and the release of prolactin. There are at least three other nerves that insert into the pelvic region including the vagus nerve, which is directly related to the sympathetic and parasympathetic systems. It's my supposition that orgasms that primarily stimulate the vagal nerve are associated with the more tidal, full body orgasmic experience, and have a gentler and more sustained endocrine profile.'

The different hormones produced by different kinds of orgasm is another area that none of the schools teaching sexuality seem to agree on. To ejaculate or not to ejaculate? What are the different influences on your health and energy levels of more sex or less sex or different types of sex? I'd need another three books to answer these questions even half satisfactorily.

I write to Nicole about the fact that some other schools are teaching a programme where they ask women not to touch the clitoris for the first six months. She writes,

'That's a little crazy as the clitoris reaches all the way back into the pussy. My experience has been that my whole pussy swells with OMing. Having said that, I would go with whatever programme they are running and follow the instructions 100% before drawing any conclusions because they likely have a different entry point.'

Nicole's advice – whatever course you are doing, do that 100% – makes sense as hopefully these are just starting points leading to the same neural pathways. But it does amuse me that, of the different sexuality training schools, some say 'stroke the external clitoris' and others say 'don't stroke the external clitoris'. The second promises more profound experiences if we explore leaving the external clitoris alone. So choose your pleasure.

So where does this leave us? To return again to my spiritual sources (with apologies to any of you that find the juxtaposition of matters of vibratory stimulation and classical texts just a little too immediate), the Buddhist *Kālāma Sutta* advises us,

'Don't believe in anything simply because you have heard it.' Or read it. Not here or even in a 'scientific study'. Look at the nonsense that we, and particularly women, have been told about their sexuality by 'scientific studies' over the years. Also, as Naomi Wolf points out, women are different. Some have more nerve endings in one area and some others. So the only way to test all this for sure is to get horizontal and explore pleasure. You have a lifetime to play. Sure beats watching TV and most straight men, or if you prefer, most gay women, will be only too willing to support you in your research.

Ecstasy on East 30th Street

Now, finally, and with apologies for the delay – back to the breath. Hooray.

I managed to go to New York in what was officially the coldest winter since they started the recording of weather temperatures in 1870. Stepping out of the apartment to a temperature of -70 degrees C was something that I'd never known. One day I stepped out with my hair still slightly wet from washing it and looked down only minutes later to see that it had frozen. The government had officially advised everyone to stay indoors and those that did venture out covered their faces giving you the curious impression that everyone was about to rob a bank. One day I stepped out and looked for a cab but after about ten minutes of waiting I understood that my body temperature was falling faster than I'd realized. I stepped into a hotel, ordered a coffee and asked them to call me a cab. The temperatures really were that dramatic. Niagara Falls froze. New York which, as you know, normally never stops, was curiously silent.

But in the room where Barbara Carrellas was taking her 'Breath and Energy Orgasm' workshop at New York's trendy centre for all things weird and wonderful, the 'Open Centre', heating was pumping out and layers of clothing were being shed. But hooray, not all the layers.

'This workshop contains no nudity and you will not be asked to reveal anything about your sex lives,' she said. How sweet are those words to my ears.

Barbara looks just as quirky and adorable in real life as she does on YouTube. She's a tiny five foot nothing, has bleached white hair dipped in bright pink; and is wearing a multi-coloured psychedelic dress. I suppose she's actually just what you'd expect an American teacher of sexuality to look like.

She is the author of several books, among them *Urban Tantra* and *Ecstasy is Necessary* and has been teaching sexuality since the 1980s.

'This is a look at what erotic energy can do. It's about the breath and the self, a heart-centred spiritual version of sex which re-defines what we mean by sexuality,' she says.

I settle down comfortably and examine my fellow attendees. There seemed to be about 17 men, 20 or so women and a few who (to steal a line from *Kinky Boots*) 'haven't yet made up their mind'). There's a woman on my left who appears to be wearing a kind of tent, has a partially-shaven head and gold-and-black ear-rings that go down to her breasts. Another woman has dreads down to her bum, which she seems to have difficulty managing.

'I'm a dom,' she says. I look blank.

'A professional dominatrix.' Of course. I knew that.

'I'm exploring how I can combine my work with tantra.' As you do.

Barbara starts her introduction.

'If you're terrified today and you showed up anyway – yayyyy for you. This is a difficult time of year. This kind of work is more popular in the spring.'

She fills us in briefly on how she got into this.

'In the 1980s a group of us were trying to meet the needs of those affected by AIDS. We formed a healing circle. We were looking for some spiritual relief but the question remained, "What are we going to do about sex?" We needed a way for people to express their sexuality that wasn't going to expose them to the virus. So we started to explore Eastern forms of sexuality. We wanted to find a way that anyone could have sex safely, but this became a spiritual and erotic practice that saved my life. The power of the breath inside us can change just about everything.'

She has my attention.

'I am not an expert in ancient traditional tantra. I don't pretend to be channeling any great mother spirit, and I'm not a guru so please don't make me into one.'

I love this.

'Now, let's go around the room and can you briefly tell us your intention today.'

Different voices from the room.

'My intention is simply to breathe and to be present with my breath.'

'I'm fighting cancer and I want to learn about the breath as I want all the ammunition I can get.'

'I'm here to have fun.'

'I'm here to increase my awareness of energy.'

'I want to expand my understanding of the healing nature of sexuality.'

A man sitting next to his partner said, 'I want to have more and better sex with him.'

'I want to work out how I can include this in my dark tantra practice.'

The idea of incorporating what I learn today into a 'dark tantra practice' is very appealing. I wish I had one somehow. I play safe and say, 'I'm here to learn about the breath.'

Barbara says,

'In sex, it's particularly important to be in the present – not in the past or the future,' she reminds us again. 'If you're in the past, you're thinking, "Will it be as good as last time?" If you're in the future, you might be thinking, "I wonder if I'm going to come?" When you focus on your breath, you come into the present moment. You jump right into the middle of the fire, into the heart of the experience so that you can go through it totally.'

We always, whether in any kind of spiritual practice or any kind of sexual practice it seems, use the breath to bring us present.

Going on with her personal story we learn that Barbara moved from teaching on the East Coast to working in Australia.

'It's easier to do tantric work in a country founded by convicts than it is in one founded by puritans.'

She jumps around from teaching to personal story and back again.

'Sex is an energy you allow rather than an action that you

do. Just let go and let the life force do you.'

I scribble notes frantically.

'It's remarkable how so much of the energy created during sex has nothing to do with the genitals. So many of the other things that we do when we are having sex build up the energy.'

Barbara uses a simple analogy that I hadn't heard this year. When she was a child she learnt how to take her bike apart to find out how it works.

'... in the same way there are various parts that make up good sex and we need to understand the components.'

This is what I have found so bewildering this year. Everywhere I have gone, all the books I have read, they all seem to have one part of the bike. They can all explain how their bit works but they may never even mention another important piece. I remember a long time ago I met Nityama, a tantric teacher, who talks a lot about the importance of women making noise. Apart from the fact that many of us live in small buildings with other people through thin walls, making noise is just one tiny part of the whole.

I've read books this year with whole chapters dedicated to the need to exercise the pelvic floor muscles or, as in slow sex, a whole book dedicated to understanding the clitoris. I did workshops with Shakti Tantra that seemed to place huge value for women in overcoming our inhibitions and learning genuine sexual expression. Then there's everything that I learnt from Alexey about touch, listening and making love with sex. And here I am today doing a whole workshop about the breath. No one seems to have taken the bike apart, shown how all the parts work and put it back together again.

'We need to learn and to understand how each of the components work to understand how the energy field builds.'

Hooray. Thank you Barbara Carrellas for that astoundingly simple piece of very necessary logic. I've learnt that, for most women, good sexual experience does not happen 'naturally'. We have to learn and understand the bike and how the parts work before we can ride. OK, enough of me, back to Barbara. She's telling us how to use thought.

'Hold up your little finger and imagine breathing into the little finger of your dominant hand, as if it were a third lung.' We breathe and imagine this.

'Now imagine filling it up with any colour you like. Now imagine it has a whole universe inside your finger.'

My finger starts to feel warm. It's unaccustomed to having a universe inside it.

'<u>The more you breathe the more you feel</u>,' she says. That's important. Underline it. Write it down. Star it in the margin or something. Highlight, write on the book, anything. Just remember those eight words. Just to make sure you do I've taken the liberty of underlining it for you myself.

We put down our buzzy fingers.

'You are going to learn to fill your whole body with life force energy. If you hold your breath when you are heading toward an orgasm you are limiting the amount of "fuel" you'll have to journey into that orgasm. You want to fill yourself completely.'

Now breathe. Take three deep breaths now. As you read. Please.

'Want to become a breath terrorist?' Barbara smiles 'Try this. When you are in a lift take some deep breaths and make a big sigh on the exhales. Watch how it totally freaks some people out.'

Ha ha ha. I love it. Why should the sound of people breathing make people so uncomfortable?

Barbara says that we often stop breathing during erotic encounters of one kind or another. She suggests that we ask our partners to remind us. Even better, perhaps, is just to breathe fully yourself and let them follow your breath.

Then she gives us the full talk on the importance of the pelvic floor muscles and ensures that I never again call the squeezing of the pubococcygeus muscle a 'Kegel'.

'I am so tired of the 20th-century phenomenon of white male doctors naming erotic techniques that women have known about for thousands of years after themselves. I'm over it.'

OK. We owe Dr Kegel a lot, but she has a point.

The next part of the bike she tells us about is the voice and how different pitches relate to different chakras (or if you're not a chakra person different parts of the body). Lots of this goes way over my head but I understand that the energy we are 'breathing in through our base chakra' (or between the legs if you prefer) has a low note with it and, as we breathe and imagine the energy travelling up the body, we make higher notes.

To practise she has us all imagine that we are making a porn movie and can't afford voiceover artists so we have to play all the parts ourselves. All at once we all do porn movie sound effects – from low grunt sounds to high-pitched squeals. Then laugh a lot. Then do more porn movie sound effects.

'Oh! Oh my! Oh my God! Ahhhhh! Aghhhhh! Yes! Ohhhh! Oooooooo ... Ahhhh.'

'Making sex sounds moves a lot of energy, but it frightens some people.' No one dies or leaves the room.

'If you find, for example, that the sound is stuck at your solar plexus, just make a higher sound. It will help to draw the energy up.'

Then finally Barbara demonstrates simple movements that we may want to make while we are breathing into the 'energy orgasm'. She moves her hips up and down and moves her arms as if she is directing the energy upwards. So, in the breathing exercise we are about to do we are asked to remember the role of the mind, the breath, the pelvic floor muscles, sound and movement. And we are about to breathe ourselves into an orgasmic state with no genital stimulation. 'The point is to explore how much energy you can allow to run through you. You want it to fill you totally, not just a small area around your genitals. Now if your fingers go all tingly or even cramp up, don't worry – they won't fall off. Sometimes this happens when you first learn the breath and energy orgasm technique. It's harmless.'

An atmosphere of nervous tension suddenly fills the room. Barbara catches it and says, 'Watch your expectations. You'll be limiting your experience if you decide, for example, that this is your fast track to a meeting with the Divine Goddess. Or, that you may as well give up now because you're a pet rock and there is no point in you doing this because you're obviously not going to experience anything at all. It's much better to just throw yourself in and see what happens, right?'

She has a pleasing logic.

'Now I'm going to give you a demonstration of a breath and energy orgasm.' Drum roll.

I can't believe that people can learn to be so uninhibited they can first learn these things and then learn to demonstrate them in a room of people.

She lies down on the floor in front of us all. And breathes and moves her arms a bit and laughs as the sensations move up her body. She's definitely not faking this. You don't build a career on something that is faked. She's somehow stimulating the nerves in her body using, as she says, a mixture of mental focus, loads of oxygen, pelvic floor squeezes, sound and movement. The sounds do not sound like a porn movie, more like the sounds of surprise you might make when your body delivers an unexpectedly good sensation. Then she laughs some more as the sounds get higher and higher, and then she changes the breathing pattern and speeds up so that she's breathing fast. Then she takes three deep breaths, and then holds her breath. There's a pause for a couple of seconds and then we see her writhing around in a state that she describes as ecstasy.

We all watch in a mixture of envy, horror, curiosity, admiration, and heaven knows how many other emotions and sensations are in the room. It's certainly hot compared to the temperatures outside.

'Let's have a break now,' says one of her assistants. 'Then later we'll come back and do this ourselves.'

So do you wish you were here with me? Or are you glad you're not? Just checking.

Come Then Go

I go out with one of the other women from the workshop. She's strikingly beautiful but I can't describe her more than that ... you're about to find out why. We chat for a while about the morning. And then, almost from nowhere, she says,

'I go to a man called Dr M. He's not a real doctor. He has a desk job during the day.'

I love a good story.

'I'm single and I got bored of masturbation. I looked round for something different. I wanted a massage with a happy ending.'

'Really? I have never met a woman in London who uses a service like this. Or I've never met one who has admitted it. It's on a massage table?'

'Never off the massage table. He's very good with his hands.'

'So, he does give you a massage then?'

'Yes. He massages you until he feels that you are relaxed enough and then he starts giving you more focused pleasure.'

I think I must look shocked. I had thought that, after this year, I was unshockable. But no.

'Does he give you any kind of instruction? I mean, ways to receive the pleasure or anything?' I vaguely wondered if this could be compared in some ways to the work I'd done with Alexey. But Alexey is clear that he's not there for 'happy endings', he's there as a coach. So this is definitely not the same.

'No instruction at all. He's just very good. He does

all kinds of things with his hands until he finds out what works for you. I've sent all my girlfriends.'

I start to laugh out loud. 'The married ones too?'

'Oh yes. The husbands think they're just having a massage.'

Ah, gullibility – thy name is man.

'Once I had orgasmed twice so we had really finished but there was ten minutes of the session left. He said, "What would you like now?" I told him whatever he wanted. He got out a large, round-shaped back vibrator, but he knew how to use it. Perhaps it was because I was in a super-sensitive state as I'd already orgasmed twice, but I had an orgasm that was about three minutes long. Non-stop. I was nearly hanging off the ceiling.'

'I've heard this year that it's possible to have a 30-minute orgasm.'

'Well, that's a new goal of mine then.'

'But how is any man in your life going to compete with Dr M?'

'The other men in my life are all happier since I've been seeing him. And I'm more confident of my body.'

'But there is no penetration?'

'It's all finger and vibrator. He's made me squirt twice and the two men I've been with since love it.'

'So, this isn't something that he taught you how to do?'

'Isabel, I didn't know that squirting existed. And since it happened with him it's happened with other men. They are very happy indeed.'

I glance at my watch and vaguely wonder if I could fit

this in before flying back to the UK. But I can't. Not that T has ever expressed any interest in seeing me squirt.

'Squirting is actually quite shocking for men. I was dating this doctor and I warned him. He said, "I'm a doctor, these things don't bother me." I asked him, "Have you ever been with a woman who squirts?"'

'No.'

'So you've never seen it?'

'No.'

'A month later it happened and he said, "Oh my God!" I had to laugh.'

'Just how much moisture was there?'

'Well, the bed had a patch about this big.' She held up her hands the size of a large dinner plate.

'Doesn't it feel a bit weird paying for massages with happy endings?'

'Yes, it does. I was very nervous at first. But a friend gave me the website and I spoke to him at length on the phone. He put me totally at my ease. So, now I don't think about it. I'm just there for the pleasure. I don't have to reciprocate or give him a blow job or spread my legs. It's all about me. I walk out of there SO happy, glowing and I can barely walk. It's the best $140 dollars I ever spend.'

• • •

But back to Barbara's ecstatic breath orgasm.

When we get back to the room it is in semi darkness. 'Find a space where you can lay down easily and extend your legs without touching anyone.'

I lie down and begin to breathe in the way that she instructs us. 'Breathe in through your mouth gently, not forcing the breath, but taking in as much air as you can. Just relax and breathe out naturally with an "ahh" sound.'

As far as I can work out what's happening here – it's because you are not pausing between one breath and another, as we do naturally, you are oxygenating the blood to an unusual balance. This has a very weird effect on the body. I squeezed my now-toned pelvic floor muscles. I breathed with her instructions. I moved my hips up and down to increase the energy. I visualized energy entering with the breath and rising up through my body. Women and men around me are doing the same but I'm really not very aware of them. I'm too surprised by the hot sensation that is building in my body.

'Don't forget to make sound.' Barbara is one of many teachers who teach that climax can be more intense when you open the throat and make sound. Barbara holds the mike and instructs us. I'm good at making low sounds. I'm good at making middle-range sounds, but not too good at the high sounds. I can hear her instructions.

'Enjoy the in-breath. Relax the jaw. Squeeze your pelvic muscles.' I go on breathing. I breathe in and let go easily and breathe in again until my whole body's singing. This must have gone on for about 20 or 30 minutes. I'm thrusting my hips in the air next to the gay male couple. I hope no one who reads this book accuses me of being inhibited. My hands and feet are tingling. My head feels light.

I go on and on breathing this way and I seem to be developing a whole new relationship with my body. I don't feel disassociated – I feel very much inside the body, but at the same time I'm not there. It's no longer as if I'm doing the breathing but as if the breathing has taken over. Mooji's question, 'Who is breathing you?' seems more relevant than ever. There's a life force here that 'I' (that is the created personality that has the name Isabel) really have nothing to do with.

'Breathe in fully. Relax. Breathe in fully. Relax.'

'Now ...' she says, 'we are going to take 30 fuller, faster breaths. Fuller, faster. In, out. In, out. In, out.' It's like pumping. I even remember to pump my pelvic floor muscles at the same time. Then she asks us to take three really full deep breaths. (How weird is this?) She says, 'Now, hold!' I hold my breath and push my bum into the floor, tense my pelvic muscles, tense my abdominal muscles. I extend my legs and push my hands down on the floor as she's shown us.

'And hold. And hold. For ten seconds, 11, 12, keep squeezing, 13, 14, 15. Then release. Now just relax and do nothing.'

I don't pretend to understand what's going on here or how it works. But it feels as if my body expands. Not in the way that I imagine a 'full body' orgasm would feel from genital stimulation, this is different. This is my body singing internally. This is heat and a feeling of pleasure that is vibrating in my body at some high pitch. My hands and feet are tingling so much they feel as if they are going to explode. I feel hot and pulsing and more alive than I ever remember feeling. And there is a feeling of astounding sweetness about it. Sweetness that somehow goes around my body and does, unexpectedly, also light up my genitals internally. It's intense.

What do we call a feeling of bliss like this? I think that, just as Barbara calls it, I'd have to call it ecstasy. It's not shared with another – which is the way I'd prefer to be experiencing this – but it's certainly the most intense physical feeling of pleasure that I've ever had. My whole body is pulsating. Weird. Around me women are laughing and making sounds of pleasure. And we haven't even taken off our clothes.

If this is the impact of just one of the bike parts, then it's certainly been underestimated. I've read whole books on sexuality this year where the breath hasn't even been mentioned. And this is free, doesn't spread disease, you don't get pregnant and you don't even need a partner.

But I haven't forgotten that my quest is about finding ways to make my sexuality work best with a partner. Neither has Barbara.

'That's an exercise in the exploration of energy with no partner and with no genital stimulation. Now ...' she smiles at her room of blissed-out beings, 'If you were to combine that with genital stimulation and a person that you love can you imagine where you'd go then?'

Touché.

Happy Endings

So, now here I am back in London. And it feels like spring. It's not spring, quite yet, but it will be soon. The snowdrops I planted last year are beginning to peep little green shoots through the cold earth. I can wear my favourite gloves that have no fingers in them and I can get into bed without a hot water bottle. Well, that's on the nights that T isn't there.

I know what you are wondering. You're wondering how all that I've learnt works out in my relationship. Is this journey going to end with a big sex scene where I manage, seamlessly, to incorporate everything into one graphic, simultaneous 30-minute multi-orgasmic experience with T where the bed collapses with exhaustion and the neighbours call the police to complain about the noise?

Were you waiting for the climax? I told you, didn't I? It's not about the climax.

This has been one of those journeys where at the beginning I knew nothing and at the end I still know nothing. But I know more about what I know nothing about. We have some fun ideas of ways we can learn. And I hope you've enjoyed the journey with me. But please don't write to me for sex advice because, as you see, I don't have any. I hope, though, that the reading has been pleasurable.

The trouble with climaxes, as Nicole says, is that they tend to end the play. And in life there are never really any endings. After whatever it is that we do in bed, that we want to be enriching and sustaining for both partners, as Alexey says, we go to sleep, then we wake up and everything goes on. The day after my return from the US I had an appointment with Clare who is testing the renewed progress of my pelvic floor muscles. (After Barbara's workshop, never again to be called 'Kegels'.) Clare was not too impressed.

'Still a bit sluggish aren't they?'

'Sluggish?'

'We want the muscles to tighten totally and relax totally. That's why we don't recommend doing these exercises with anything inside like a vibrator or those metal things that you have to squeeze. We want the muscles to come together completely but also to be able to relax. Also we don't want the muscles to just be pulled up. We want them "up and forward". Can you feel here?'

I squeeze even harder.

'Yes, that's better. But you've also got to learn never to hold your breath when you're squeezing and not to use your abs at all. Next time we'll put you on the biofeedback machine. Now that you understand the different muscle groups better you'll benefit from seeing the biofeedback. But this will take six months you know.'

'Six months?'

'It's like any exercise programme. You can't expect your muscles to change shape in a matter of weeks. If you go to the gym you're not going to change your body shape without real hard work. This is the same.'

'I see.'

'But are you noticing any change?'

I honestly think that I am. When T and I last made love I'm sure I felt him inside me in a way that I've never felt him before. I felt as if I could feel the shape of him better. I may have made this up and it may have been just my imagination – but I honestly don't think so because it was unexpected. I hadn't been looking for a feeling like that ... so why would I imagine it? T hasn't been doing any exercises to increase his size – so if I can feel him better then it can only be because I'm more toned. I explain all this to Clare.

'So, it does genuinely seem to be increasing my pleasure – even if they are still, "sluggish." Great word, Clare. And after I've been doing these exercises five times a day? "Must try harder."'

'They're not that bad compared to some of the women I see. Sometimes they can't register a movement on the machine or on my finger. I see lots of women here that have never had orgasms of any kind.'

'Not of any kind at all?'

'Nope. Women often tell me this.'

Now maybe the women who end up going to see Clare are women who have never toned these muscles and so therefore are a group of women least likely to have had orgasms. But all the same ... come on, women! Pleasure isn't supposed to be an optional extra in life. There are so many ways to learn. So many courses, doctors, teachers, even – as I was hearing in New York – masseurs that offer 'happy endings'. Even though it's not about the climax, it's good to have a happy ending sometimes or to at least have that possibility. It's not about the man. It's about taking responsibility for your own pleasure. You'll be dead soon.

I recommend that everyone move pleasure up the agenda of what's important. Because pleasure (I say radical things sometimes) feels good and can make you happier. And if you're happier you'll be a better mother, father, wife, husband, son, daughter, lover or friend. You'll simply be better to be around. Now which path you go down, that's up to you. As long as it's adult and consenting and everyone is truthful to everyone else. Truth, for me, is an essential part of love and love is what's it all about. Sex is just one more way to express love. 'And is Dr M expressing love?' you may ask rather cynically. Well, I've never met him. But I'd say, 'Yes'.

It's not the fairy-tale kind of love. Not I-own-you-so-I'm-clingy-and-jealous-and-I-want-you-all-to-myself-for-ever-and-better-not-touch-another-person-ever-or-you'll-have-to-lie-about-it kind of love. But – and you can laugh at me if you like – I'd say it's part of the kind of love that is in everything and everyone. It's a shame that some of the women who go to Dr M feel that they have to lie to their husbands. Some of those husbands may be having affairs and lying back. I don't judge anything anymore. But I see what Dr M does as loving. And what Alexey does and what happens at the Inns of Court at the weekends. I see love everywhere. Maybe I've done too many seminars and listened to too many spiritual teachers.

And what about my relationship with T, you ask? Am I about to give you a scene where we walk along the beach into the sunset? Endings of books are always tricky because we have such a need for a happy conclusion. Just think how satisfying it would feel if I wrote, 'T and I are going to get married, move in together, and we've been to Battersea Dogs Home to rescue a couple of unwanted hounds. And you're all invited to the romantic happy ending which will be held at ...'

I'd love to write that to give you that warm, fuzzy end-of-book feeling. And did you know that books with happy endings actually sell more? Ha ha. This is fine for writers of fiction and is the reason that some writers of non-fiction make them up anyway. I'm not making anything up. I like real life. It's harsher but true. It's wakes us up. It's well ... real. And real life is often a little more complicated than fiction.

Even when life does give fairy-tale endings, they are really joyful beginnings, aren't they? There is a real relationship and a real sex life to sustain and to enjoy in the years that follow. And that's what this book has been about. It's about after happily ever after.

I have no idea about the future any more than you do. There is only today. You know this.

'And "T"?' you enquire. So I ask him.

'How was this year for you? I remember at the beginning of the year you said that you already knew everything.'

'Hmmmm. Yes. Well, now I know a little less'

'Or maybe we know a little about what we know nothing about?'

'I think that's the safer conclusion. And the one with the most potential. Do you have any plans for Friday night?'

It's been four amazing seasons. And hopefully you know that with each, er, book, it's the joy of the ride that counts.

I hope you've enjoyed this one and learnt some useful stuff that maybe one sunny day or cosy night you can share with someone. Thanks for listening. A good listener is also a good lover, remember. Write me to me online or on my Facebook page. May your bed be always warm – whether it's a lover or a hot water bottle that warms it. Keep breathing. And thank you.

xxx

www.isabellosada.com

NOTES

1   You can see the altar at:
    http://www.pinterest.com/isabellosada/sensation/
2   Women's courses at www.shaktitantra.co.uk
3   Song lyrics by Libby Roderick.
4   The first ever TED talk to go viral from Jill Bolte Taylor:
    www.ted.com/talks/jillboltetaylorspowerfulstrokeofinsight
5   Uta Demontis, *The Jade Egg Practice – Sexercises for your
    Love Muscle* (Uta Demontis, 2015)
6   Visit Deborah's site to find out more: http://
    www.isismedia.org
7   http://pinterest.com/isabellosada/ecstasy/
8   www.manawa.co.uk
9   Find details for the workshop at: http://
    www.shaktitantra.co.uk/mixed
10 See the Sensation Pinterest page again – there is a pencil
    drawing of the correct position for OMing there: http://
    www.pinterest.com/isabellosada/sensation/
11 The OM/OneTaste websites:
    UK – www.turnonbritain.co.uk,
    US and International – www.onetaste.us
12 'If I Didn't Have You' by Tim Minchin.
    www.youtube.com/TimMinchin/If
13 www.sophiawallace.com/cliteracy-100-natural-laws
14 www.isabellosada.com/isabel-recommends/poems/
    Mary-Oliver
15 http://anandawave.tantramassagen.de/ausbildung-
    seminare

16 www.tantrictherapy.co.uk

17 http://www.nityama.com/blog

18 http://www.sashacobra.com

19 www.rachaelis.com

20 www.greatwallofvagina.co.uk/home

21 http://www.lucyslusciousrawchocolate.co.uk

22 http://www.haskeladamson.blogspot.co.uk

23 If you, or anyone you know, suffer from vaginismus there is a wealth of information at www.vaginismus.com or please do go to your GP.

24 www.shesaidboutique.com

25 Bondage/Discipline Dominance/Submission Sadomasochism

26 www.dossieeaston.com

27 www.drewlawson.co

28 Anne Novak, Breath of Fire (Kundalini Yoga as taught by Yogi Bhajan ®). See https://www.youtube.com/watch?v=V86Xao9bcRI

29 www.buteyko.com

30 Breath & Energy Orgasm/Barbara Carrellas. See https://www.youtube.com/watch?v=OEznv88LfbY

FURTHER READING

There is a lot of reading out there. Here are some books that I read this year in alphabetical order by author:

The Art of Sexual Ecstasy by Margo Anand (Tarcher, 1989)
If you want to study tantra in detail and have time that you can dedicate to developing real skill, then this book is an essential guide.

How to Think More about Sex by Alain de Botton
(Macmillan, 2012)
He's fantastically weird.

Ecstasy is Necessary: A Practical Guide by Barbara Carrellas
(Hay House, 2012)
Very 'American' (for US readers, read very 'Californian')
but excellent if you wish to learn to take more erotic risks in your life. Excellent on values, how to establish and expand boundaries, communicate wisely and expand what Barbara would call your ecstatic life experience – which she doesn't limit to sexuality.

The Multi-Orgasmic Couple by Mantak Chia (HarperCollins, 2000)
This book is written from the male perspective, but Mantak Chia is one of the leaders of the field and is especially good with practices for men on how to separate orgasm from ejaculation.

Slow Sex by Nicole Daedone (Grand Central, 2011)
The textbook in case you'd like to try Orgasmic Meditation (OMing) at home. Also some wonderful writing on what women want from men and what men want from women.

The Jade Egg Practice: Sexercises for Your Love Muscle by Uta Demontis
Liven up your PC workouts or your yoga practise by combining what you do with some of Uta's jade egg exercises. Life is short after all:-)

The Brain that Changes Itself by Dr Norman Doidge (Viking, 2006)
This is the book about neuro-plasticity that I refer to. Not a hard read. Although not specifically about sexuality, this book explains how the brain and the body learn to re-wire themselves. This is why practise in any new experience of pleasure works. Whether your method of learning is more like Nicole's, more like Alexey's, with just your partner at home or if you want to go off and explore. Also inspiring if you know anyone who has had a stroke or suffered brain damage of any kind.

The Vagina Monologues by Eve Ensler (Virago, 2001)
I'd already seen the play some years ago but it didn't impact like reading the book. If you or your daughters haven't read this, I'd say it's pretty essential education for women. And men too.

Fear of Flying by Erica Jong (Martin Secker & Warburg, 1973)
Finally got around to reading this 1970s epic, as I was
curious to see what all the fuss had been about. It's
an enjoyable and easy read. Rather what today we'd call
'chick-lit' about a gutsy New Yorker who runs away from
her husband to search for 'the zipless fuck'.

A General Theory of Love by Thomas Lewis, Fari Amini
and Richard Lannon (Knopf Doubleday, 2000)
Recommended by Nicole Daedone and popular in the
OM community, this challenging book by three eminent
psychiatrists explains what is meant by 'the limbic
connection', how it works, can be trained and the
implications of this in our lives.

I'd recommend to anyone who wants to understand
why they may fall in love with the 'wrong' people. My only
regret is that it is rather too good on explaining the nature
of the problem and thinner on what can be done about it,
other than to have traditional therapy – but even that comes
with a warning that you need to find a sane and balanced
therapist. But good reading if you struggle to understand
your own behaviour.

Tantra: The Cult of the Feminine by Andre Van Lysebeth
(Red Wheel, 2002)
A little lengthy, and the late Andre used far too many
exclamation marks, but a wonderful overview of the cult of
the feminine in history and includes an entire chapter on
how to strengthen the sexual muscles. A little hard to find

and expensive but a must-read for anyone with a genuine interest in the history of tantric practice.

The Great Wall of Vagina by Jamie McCartney (Jamie McCartney, 2011)
This book contains not only breath-taking photos of the vulva casts that make up Jamie's 'Great Wall' but the story of the creation of the Wall and the responses of the women involved in the project.

How to Be a Woman by Caitlin Moran (Penguin Random House, 2011)
I would make this book compulsory reading for every woman under 30 and recommended optional reading for women aged 30–100. The conclusions of her chapter on porn are so brilliant that I would like to have quoted about three pages in full. Also a fun and easy read and will make you laugh. In the unlikely event of you not having read it yet ... I recommend it.

The Diary of Anaïs Nin: Volume One 1931–1934, Volume Two 1934–1939, Volume Three 1939–1944
If you want erotic inspiration for your life, immerse yourself in Anaïs Nin. Here is a taster ... a page of quotes from her. www.thoughtcatalog.com/christine-stockton/2013/09/41-completely-badgirl-anais-nin-quotes

Girls & Sex by Peggy Orenstein. (HarperCollins, 2016)
When people say 'this book saved a life' it's usually

an exaggeration. I can honestly say that I put my own daughter's life and happiness in danger when she was a teenager by not having read this book. If you have a daughter, you simply must read this book. You'll understand why I express this so strongly when you've read it. It's not a fun read. But it's very important. Especially for parents of girls.

Tantra: The Supreme Understanding by Osho (Rebel Publishing, 1997)
No matter what your thoughts are about Osho, he can explain the more esoteric aspects of tantric thought better than anyone. This book is a series of talks that he gave on Tilopa's (988–1069) 'The Song of the Mahamudra', which is a teaching from Tantric Buddhism.

Tantric Orgasm for Women by Diana Richardson (Destiny Books, 2004)
As you may remember, this is one I haven't read. But if you want to know what a 'Valley Orgasm' is apparently it's all in here. Write and let me know ...

Yoni Massage: Awakening Female Sexual Energy by Michaela Riedl (Destiny Books, 2009)
If this subject has confused or interested you then you can read more about it here (she also talks about the Breath Orgasm, which she calls 'The Big Draw'). Or, of course, you can go to Germany and learn more.

My Stroke of Insight by Jill Bolte Taylor (Penguin Books, 2008)
Not specifically about sex unless you believe, as Alexey teaches, that sex and love are all about energy, in which case this book will help you understand what Jill means by the phrase 'please be responsible for the energy you bring to this place'. With all the language centres in her brain damaged, when someone came to visit her in hospital all Jill experienced was their energy. A great read too.

A New Earth by Eckhart Tolle (Viking, 2005)
If all that conversation about 'ego' and 'Advaita' and us not being 'our conditioned self' lost you, then you may like to read *A New Earth* – or *The Power of Now*. Great spiritual reading if you don't know how to switch your thoughts off or to realize that they don't matter.

The Kama Sutra by Vatsyayana
Am delighted to discover the charm in this 2,000-year-old Hindu text. A surprisingly small amount of this sutra is about sex. A lot of it also has other useful practical advice such as how to keep your harem happy, how to break into the king's harem to make love to his wives and how to get as much money out of your clients as possible if you're a professional.

Vagina by Naomi Wolf (Virago, 2013)
An important book which is both extensively researched and courageously personal. Ultimately I'm not sure that

I agree with Naomi on some points but it's a very important read, especially on the subject of the history and subjugation of women's sexuality.

Promiscuities: An Opinionated History of Female Desire by Naomi Wolf (Random House, 1997)
Naomi writes about growing up as a young woman with a sex drive. I wish I could have given this book to my daughter and her friends when they were all 16. If you have a daughter you may like to read this book. And if you are between 15 and 25, I recommend that you read it yourself.

Introduction to Tantra: The Transformation of Desire by Lama Yeshe (Wisdom Publications, 1997)
This book is not about any tantric sexual practices but about Tantric Buddhism. If you really want to understand about desire (not just sexual desire but all desire) and how tantra teaches that you can take that energy and utilize it for your greater happiness – then the late Lama Yeshe speaks on this in his clear introduction to tantra. Then it becomes less clear.

Some Viewing

TV: *Masters of Sex*
If you didn't catch this excellent American TV series it's absolutely worth paying £2.49 an episode to watch it at home. (Please don't download illegally – people in the arts need their work supporting.) The series is about the life

of the sex research pioneers Masters and Johnson, and manages the perfect combination of drama, entertainment and genuine sexual education.

Film: *The Sessions*
Award-winning American independent drama film (2012) written and directed by Ben Lewin about a paraplegic who hires a sex surrogate to teach him about sexuality. Beautiful. www.thesessionsmovie.com

Apps

This where to obtain the NHS 'Squeezy' app:
https://itunes.apple.com/gb/app/squeezy-nhs-physiotherapy/id700740791?mt=8

'Kegel Aerobics' App with nine levels. (Good luck with level nine.)
http://kegelaerobics.com

Websites

There are many but http://www.ohmygodyes.com is especially good.

Short Word of Warning

I want to alert you to the fact that, as with all human potential and personal development work, some courses that teach sexuality can be expensive.

Some of them use 'hard sell' techniques for their higher level courses that I'm ashamed of.

Please never sign up for any course, of any kind, at and introduction event no matter how great the 'discount' that is on offer if you do so.

NEVER borrow money to do a course. Never take out a loan. Never get into debt to take a workshop. There is no course on earth that is worth getting into debt for.

For example – the beauty of the OM experience is in the actual practise. This can be explored with my book, Nicole's book, a pot of their One Taste Lube (because it's the right viscosity) and a loving and curious partner. Maybe a private lesson if you get stuck.

But 'One Taste' (like many businesses) offer a wide range of courses which are outside the price range of most bank accounts. I'll say it again. Please don't spend money that you don't have.

On the other hand – if you are fortunate enough to be wealthy then (in my opinion) your money would be better spent on studying sexuality for a year and buying a cheaper car – for example. Life is short and the body is designed for pleasure.

Always give careful consideration before signing up to a course or a series of courses. If in doubt send me an email or a message.

Take care of yourself.
xxx Isabel

ACKNOWLEDGEMENTS

All the people in this book are real. In rare cases I have changed someone's name to protect his or her identity, but most people appear as themselves so I would like to thank everyone who is mentioned in these pages and has played a part.

Inspiration for a more profound level of understanding about sexuality comes primarily, for me, from Hilary Spenceley, at Shakti Tantra, whose lifetime of dedication to teaching and liberating both women and men from everything that stands between them and the full enjoyment and celebration of their own pleasure is profoundly beautiful and has inspired all those that have come into contact with her. Special thanks are also due to Sue Newsome and Martin Hellawell, also at Shakti Tantra, for their patience with me. I am so grateful to these three for their skill and generosity in allowing me to describe so much of their material. Thanks to all the brave souls in the women's workshops and the couples' workshops. I have huge admiration for everyone who does this work.

Thank you very much to Rachel Cherwitz, Rachael Hemsi, Maya Block, Justyna Kucharska, Elena Maxwell, Marc Quin, Adam Jacobowitz, Claudia Melli, Kapil Gupta, Chris Eadie, Clouds L. de Narvaez, Michael Silbert and all the other inspiring and wonderful beings I met in the OM community for your encouragement along the way. Especially to Nicole Daedone for her joyful courage and love of life, to Justine Dawson who just gets everything right in a most extraordinary way, to Ken Blackman for proving the teachings are real and to Jeff Ridenour for the quality of his practice. Thanks to Emma Jane Thompson for making The Golden Gate Bridge ours forever.

Other teachers and fellow pupils of sexuality on the path that I'd like to thank are, Alexey Kuzmin for existing – I wish I could have heard all that you teach when I was 18; thank you for your profound kindness and generosity during this process. Thanks to Mike (no relation) Lousada for his knowledge, to Drew Lawson for answering so many of my questions, to Jovanna Desmarais for her humour, and to Angela Sabine and Hanna Steinschlag for being truly beautiful women. Thank you to Uta Demontis for sending me those three and for your commitment to teaching your material.

In Sussex, thank you to Steve and Laura Griffiths for creating the 'Love, Sex and Intimacy Fair', to Lucky and Albert for hosting, to Rachel McCoy for being delightful, to Jamie McCartney for his *Great Wall of Vagina*, to Nic Ramsey for talking about PCs, and to everyone who came to my own talk on my book, *Men!*, one memorable evening.

Thank to Clare and her amazing boss at the Chelsea and Westminster Hospital and – although I know it's a lot of people to thank – to anyone and everyone who works for the NHS. Thank you to my astounding dentist for giving me her story, to Saby Harmony for allowing the inclusion of the details of her events and to Linda for explaining to me about Kundalini. Thank you to Barbara Carrellas for permission to write about my experience in her workshop.

In the publishing world I would like to thank two agents, Julia Cameron and Jane Graham Maw, for their hard work and confidence in the book. At Watkins, thanks to Michael Mann for being wonderful, to James Spackman for asking, my editor Kate Latham for her patience, my publisher Jo Lal for backing the book from the start and to Etan Ilfeld for making everything possible. Also to Vicky Hartley – for being Vicky Hartley.

Most especial thanks to Caroline Sanderson who read the book twice, as a manuscript, believed in the work when I doubted it myself and spoke words of wisdom and inspiration at moments when I most needed to hear them. I would also like to thank Carole Tonkinson for her constant kindness and for picking me up on more than one occasion and speaking to me as if I was a sane person at moments when I didn't feel like one. I owe a profound debt of gratitude to these two extraordinary women.

Closer to home I'd like to thank my daughter Emily for her tolerance (who wants a mother who writes a book about sexuality?), Gala and Jane for reading the book in manuscript and for all thoughtful comments and suggestions; Polly and Daisy for listening to me; my guardian angels JJM and CM for making it possible for me to get to San Francisco and New York; and to the man I've called 'T' for absolutely everything. Rare is a man whose passion for love and life results in him saying 'Yes, please' – whatever adventure is suggested. I'm privileged to know you. Thank you very much.

Finally, I'd like to thank that core bunch of loyal readers who have read all the books from *The Battersea Park Road to Enlightenment* through Tibet and the Amazon to this one, especially those on my Facebook, Twitter and Instagram pages who offer words of encouragement, write reviews and buy copies of my books for everyone you know. A career as an author is not always easy but the loyalty, wisdom and generous friendliness of readers makes the job a joy. You are too many to list by name – but if you are reading this then you are now undoubtedly one of them. Thank you.

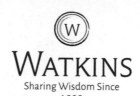

WATKINS

Sharing Wisdom Since
1893

The story of Watkins dates back to 1893, when the scholar of esotericism John Watkins founded a bookshop, inspired by the lament of his friend and teacher Madame Blavatsky that there was nowhere in London to buy books on mysticism, occultism or metaphysics. That moment marked the birth of Watkins, soon to become the home of many of the leading lights of spiritual literature, including Carl Jung, Rudolf Steiner, Alice Bailey and Chögyam Trungpa.

Today, the passion at Watkins Publishing for vigorous questioning is still resolute. Our wide-ranging and stimulating list reflects the development of spiritual thinking and new science over the past 120 years. We remain at the cutting edge, committed to publishing books that change lives.

DISCOVER MORE . . .

Read our blog

Watch and listen to
our authors in action

Sign up to
our mailing list

JOIN IN THE CONVERSATION

WatkinsPublishing @watkinswisdom

watkinsbooks watkinswisdom watkins-media

Our books celebrate conscious, passionate, wise and happy living.
Be part of the community by visiting

www.watkinspublishing.com